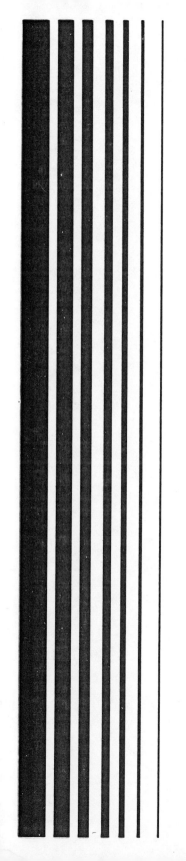

SUICIDE
IN THE
ELDERLY

CONTRIBUTORS

Dan G. Blazer II
Soo Borson
Mary Lou Melville
Richard C. Veith

SUICIDE IN THE ELDERLY

A Practitioner's Guide to Diagnosis and Mental Health Intervention

Nancy J. Osgood, Ph.D.
Virginia Commonwealth University/
Medical College of Virginia
Richmond, Virginia

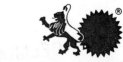

AN ASPEN PUBLICATION®
Aspen Systems Corporation
Rockville, Maryland
Royal Tunbridge Wells
1985

Library of Congress Cataloging in Publication Data

Osgood, Nancy J.
Suicide in the elderly

"An Aspen publication."
Includes index.
1. Geriatric psychiatry. 2. Suicide. I. Title.
RC451.4.A5084   1985   618.97'689   85-1319
ISBN: 0-87189-088-7

Managing Editor: M. Eileen Higgins
Editorial Services: Jane Coyle
Printing and Manufacturing: Debbie Collins

Library of Congress Catalog Card Number: 85-1319
ISBN: 0-87189-088-7

Printed in the United States of America

1 2 3 4 5

This book is lovingly dedicated

to my friend and husband, Ray

Table of Contents

Preface

After a serious suicide attempt Peter Putnam (1959) wrote:

> The extreme negation of life (suicide) is the sole positive control over life, the only irrevocable decision a man can impose upon his future. Through complete selfishness, it confers utter selflessness . . . . although it is a symptom of a diseased mind, it is entirely rational. To the individual living in perfect isolation, it is the only logical escape from the suffering isolation. (p. 26)

If the suicide statistics available for the United States accurately reflect the pulse of the American people, then it seems that many of us share Putnam's sentiments regarding suicide. In 1983 someone committed suicide every 19 minutes in this country; 27,860 individuals willfully chose to take their own lives. The national suicide rate for 1982 was 12 per 100,000 of the United States population (provisional figures based on a 10-percent sample taken by the National Center for Health Statistics) (NCHS, 1983). This figure represents a rate very similar to the 1900 suicide rate—a startling fact when we consider the lowered death rates from most major diseases since that time. For American males of all ages, suicide is the 7th leading cause of death; for American females it is the 10th leading cause of death. More importantly, suicide represents the first and leading cause of unnecessary, stigmatizing death (Yolles, 1968).

Suicide has been part of the human experience since the beginning of time. It has been discovered in primitive as well as modern societies of the world. It has variously been condemned as an immoral act and a sin, and exalted as the highest form of human behavior, giving humans control over death itself.

A voluminous literature has developed on the subject of suicide; however, we are still in no position to specify clearly the causes of suicide or to suggest effective preventives. We are able to identify some "at-risk" groups in the population based on demographic analysis. We are also able to specify various characteristics of the environment and particular personality traits that predispose an individual to commit suicide. However, we have very few good in-depth studies of completed suicides that allow us to trace the development of what Maris (1969) terms the "suicidal career" of individuals.

Suicide rates for different age groups suggest that suicide in the United States, and in most other industrialized countries for which data are available, is clearly more frequent among older than among younger persons (Atchley, 1982; Dublin, 1963; Maris, 1969; McIntosh, Hubbard, & Santos, 1981; Niccolini, 1973; Sainsbury, 1962; Weiss, 1968).

Although the oft-cited statement that the aged comprise 10 percent of the population but commit 25 percent of the suicides exaggerates the case (McIntosh et al., 1981), the positive relationship between age and suicide is essentially accurate. Researchers (McIntosh et al., 1981) who based their finding on U.S. Census figures from 1978 and on official statistics compiled by the National Center for Health Statistics in 1976 found that those aged 65 and over made up only 10.7 percent of the U.S. population but committed 17 percent of the suicides. Miller (1976), who analyzed 1975 data from the National Center for Health Statistics, notes that more than 10,000 persons aged 60 and over kill themselves each year. Data from that year revealed that those aged 60 and over represented 18.5 percent of the U.S. population but committed 23 percent of all suicides (Miller, 1979). It is thus clear that more older people kill themselves than do younger people.

Most elderly who attempt suicide are deadly serious about killing themselves. Unlike younger individuals, the elderly seldom attempt suicide as a cry for help or a means by which to get attention (Miller, 1979). According to Sendbuehler and Goldstein (1977), the ratio of completed suicides to suicide attempts for the elderly is approximately 8:1. Several studies confirm that elderly persons almost always succeed in killing themselves and rarely make attempts that fail (Gardner, Bahn, & Mack, 1964; Grollman, 1971; Kreitman, 1977; Resnik & Cantor, 1970). The elderly more often use lethal means and have less recuperative power —two possible explanations for the higher percentage of successful suicides in this age group (Batchelor & Napier, 1953; Benson & Brodie, 1975; Dublin, 1963; McIntosh et al., 1981; O'Neal, Robins, & Schmidt, 1956).

Dramatic as these figures are, they underestimate the frequency of suicide among the aged. Many such suicides are not recognized and/or reported as suicides. Compared to other age groups, the elderly can more easily take overdoses of drugs, mix drugs, fail to take life-sustaining drugs, starve themselves, drink excessively, or have fatal "accidents" (Osgood, 1982).

Although suicide in the elderly represents a major social problem, it has been virtually ignored in the United States. Attention has consistently focused on adolescent suicide, betraying our culture's emphasis on youth and devaluation of the aged. After all, if an older person commits suicide, how many will be around to mourn and feel a loss?

This book has been in the making for several years. In 1975, while employed as a research fellow at Hutchings Psychiatric Center in Syracuse, New York, I was involved in a purely academic study of suicide. The task was to examine the records of the county coroner in order to gather descriptive statistics on the number of suicides by age and sex. At some point during the study, while reading the suicide notes of different individuals of varying ages, it became apparent that many of the victims were over 60, and that many of them had lost all hope for a happy, meaningful existence. What began as a purely academic pursuit suddenly took on new personal meaning for me. I was impressed with the magnitude of the problem of elderly suicide, as well as with some of the reasons offered by those elderly individuals who chose to take their own lives. What it means to be old in our society was highlighted in the suicide notes of those who had retired or who faced serious health or financial problems. The picture that emerged from the myriad of notes was not a pretty one. At that point in my career, although I did very little with the information I had gathered and the impressions I had formed, the seed was planted.

A few years later in 1978 I conducted a study (funded by the National Institute of Mental Health) of life in retirement communities. During the course of the study I discovered some husbands and wives whose spouses had committed suicide. I interviewed these individuals to obtain more information about the suicides. Again I was impressed with the magnitude of the problem of elderly suicide and with the conditions surrounding the deaths. Two questions kept running through my mind: Why do so many elderly individuals kill themselves? and, What can we as a society do to prevent these unnecessary deaths of our older members?

This book is written for all those working with the elderly who want to know why the elderly are more likely to commit suicide and how to recognize and help such individuals before they choose the final solution to their problems. Its purpose is to examine in detail the problem of elderly suicide. The emphasis is on identifying potential suicide victims in the elderly population and on specifying appropriate assessment techniques and intervention strategies that can be employed by professionals working with the elderly.

In the Introduction, we present an overview of theoretical and conceptual models and explanations of elderly suicide. Part I of the book focuses on the detection and assessment of suicidal risk and lethality. Profiles of the "at-risk" elderly are presented. Various factors that predispose elderly individuals to kill themselves are also discussed. Particular attention is given to the impact of retirement, loss of spouse, pain, and illness. Also, assessment scales and techniques to measure depression, life satisfaction, loneliness, and stress are reviewed. Finally, the roles of the doctor, nurse, priest or rabbi, social worker, psychologist or psychiatrist, behavioral gerontologist, and other "gatekeepers" in the assessment of the suicidal potential of the elderly client are discussed.

Suicide prevention and intervention is the focus of Part II. In these chapters, we highlight several forms of therapy that have proven to be effective with the depressed and troubled elderly. Drug therapy, reminiscence or life review therapy, creative therapies (art, drama, dance, and music), and support group or peer group intervention are each discussed in detail in individual chapters.

Those working with the vulnerable elderly should possess certain personal qualities and skills and should utilize specific counseling techniques and strategies if they are to be effective. These qualities and skills are outlined in Chapter 5. Special attention is given to the techniques of intervention for the bereaved. Chapter 10 focuses on how to help the elderly cope with stress and manage tension. In the final chapter, we offer some suggestions for societal changes that could help reduce the rate of elderly suicide in this country.

It is hoped that this book might in some small way help to alleviate the frustrations and anxieties of those working with the depressed, suicide-prone elderly and also to reduce the number of elderly suicides in this country.

REFERENCES

Atchley, R. C. (1982). Aging and suicide: Reflections on the quality of life. In S. G. Haynes, M. Feinlib, J. A. Ross, & L. Stallones (Eds.), *Epidemiology of aging* (NIH Publication No. 8–969, p. 158). Washington, D.C.: U. S. Department of Health and Human Services.

Batchelor, I. R. C., & Napier, M. (1953). Attempted suicide in old age. *British Medical Journal, 2,* 1186–1190.

Benson, R., & Brodie, D. (1975). Suicide by overdoses of medicines among the aged. *Journal of the American Geriatrics Society, 23,* 304–308.

Dublin, L. (1963). *Suicide.* New York: Ronald Press.

Gardner, E. A., Bahn, A. K., & Mack, M. (1964). Suicide and psychiatric care in the aging. *Archives of General Psychiatry, 10,* 547–553.

Grollman, E. (1971). *Suicide: Prevention, intervention, and postvention.* Boston: Beacon Press.

Kreitman, N. (1977). *Parasuicide.* New York: John Wiley & Sons.

Maris, R. W. (1969). *Social forces in urban suicide.* New York: Dorsey Press.

McIntosh, J. L., Hubbard, R. W., & Santos, J. F. (1981). Suicide among the elderly: A review of issues with case studies. *Journal of Gerontological Social Work, 4*(1), 63–74.

Miller, M. (1976). *Suicide among older men.* Unpublished doctoral dissertation, University of Michigan.

Miller, M. (1979). *Suicide after sixty: The final alternative.* New York: Springer.

National Center for Health Statistics. (1983). Annual summary of births, deaths, marriages, and divorces: United States, 1982. *Monthly Vital Statistics Report, 31*(13), 24.

Niccolini, R. (1973). Reading the signals for suicidal risk. *Geriatrics, 28,* 71–72.

O'Neal, P., Robins, E., & Schmidt, E. H. (1956). A psychiatric study of attempted suicide in persons over sixty years of age. *Archives of Neurological Psychiatry, 75,* 275–284.

Osgood, N. J. (1982). Suicide in the elderly: Are we heeding the warnings? *Postgraduate Medicine, 72,* 84–88.

Putnam, P. (1959). *Cast out the darkness.* London: Peter Davies.

Resnik, H. L. P., & Cantor, J. (1970). Suicide and aging. *Journal of the American Geriatrics Society, 18,* 152–158.

Sainsbury, P. (1962). Suicide in later life. *Gerontologica Clinica, 4,* 161–170.

Sendbuehler, J. M., & Goldstein, S. (1977). Attempted suicide among the aged. *Journal of the American Geriatrics Society, 25,* 245–248.

Weiss, J. M. A. (1968). Suicide in the aged. In H. L. P. Resnik (Ed.), *Suicidal behaviors: Diagnosis and management* (pp. 255–267). Boston: Little, Brown & Co.

Yolles, S. (1968). Suicide: A public health problem. In H. L. P. Resnik (Ed.), *Suicidal behaviors: Diagnosis and management* (pp. 49–56). Boston: Little, Brown & Co.

Acknowledgments

I would like to thank all those who made the completion of this book possible. First, my thanks to Drs. Mary Lou Melville, Dan Blazer, Soo Borson, and Richard C. Veith for their contributed chapters. Next, my thanks to Clinton Browne, John Damrau, and Brenda Mann, who read the manuscript and made valuable comments that improved the work. I would also like to thank John McIntosh for his support and encouragement and for the valuable information he kindly shared with me. All of my colleagues who have listened to my ideas and contributed to my knowledge and understanding about suicide deserve a word of thanks. Thanks also to Walter Norman, Marie Fleming, and Susan Griffith for their typing, proofreading, and other able assistance in the production of this work. Lastly, I am indebted to my daughter, Cressida, and my husband, Ray, for their patience and endurance during the writing of this book.

Introduction

THE CASE OF THE ELDERLY SUICIDE: CONTRIBUTING FACTORS, THEORETICAL EXPLANATIONS, AND CONCEPTUAL MODELS

In approximately the third century B.C., the well-known Roman stoic Seneca delivered the following discourse on suicide in old age:

> For this reason, but for this alone, life is not an evil—that no one is obliged to live. If life pleases you, live. If not, you have a right to return whence you came. I will not relinquish old age if it leaves my better part intact. But if it begins to shake my mind, if it destroys its facilities one by one, if it leaves me not life but breath, I will depart from the putrid or tottering edifice. I will not escape by death from disease so long as it may be healed, and leaves my mind unimpaired. I will not raise my hand against myself on account of pain, for so to die is to be conquered. But if I know that I must suffer without hope of relief, I will depart, not through fear of the pain itself, but because it prevents all for which I would live (Lecky, 1869, pp. 219–220).

Through the centuries, suicide has generally been philosophically condoned as more appropriate for the old, especially those who are physically ill or suffering intense pain, than for members of any other age group. Pliny the Elder considered the existence of poisonous herbs proof of a kindly Providence because it allowed people to die painlessly and quickly and thus avoid the pain and sickness of old age. Zeno, the founder of Stoic philosophy, similarly advocated suicide to avoid the pain and sickness of late life; at age

98, when he fell down and pulled his toe out of joint, he hanged himself. Diogenes, the Cynic, also favored suicide among the old. He wrote, "A wise man will quit life, when oppressed with severe pain, or deprived of any of his senses, or when laboring under desperate diseases" (Dublin, 1963, p. 194).

In primitive societies, it was conventional, and occasionally obligatory, for old people to commit suicide if because of their infirmities they had become a burden on the other members of the community (Batchelor & Napier, 1953). The ancient Scythians regarded suicide as the greatest honor when they became too old for their nomadic life (Alvarez, 1972); and on the island of Cheos in Greek antiquity it was normal for the old and the weak to commit suicide (Baqucher, 1979). Institutionalized suicide of the elderly among the Eskimos is a well-attested fact.

Today, in the United States and other westernized, industrialized nations of the world, the suicide rate is highest for the old. In the following pages, we review the relevant literature on demographic factors in geriatric suicide and discuss various social, psychological, physical, and other contributing factors that precipitate suicide among the aged. Theoretical explanations and conceptual models are presented to explain and interpret findings from a wide variety of studies in different disciplines. Finally, a model of elderly suicide that integrates all of these factors and perspectives is presented.

DEMOGRAPHIC FACTORS

Suicide is indeed more prevalent among the elderly; however, certain segments of the elderly population are more likely to commit suicide than others. Specifically, elderly white males are the most vulnerable. This section reviews major findings from studies that have examined the roles of sex, race, marital status, social class and occupation, and the living environment in suicide among the elderly.

Sex

In all age groups, suicide rates are significantly higher for males than for females (Bromley, 1966; Burvil, 1972; Dublin, 1963; Durkheim, 1951). So pronounced is this trend that Dublin (1963) has referred to suicide as a "masculine type of behavior." The disparity of male and female suicide rates is more pronounced for the elderly than for any other age group.

Suicide among the elderly has consistently proven to be more prevalent among males (Atchley, 1980; Bock, 1972; Botwinick, 1973; Burvil, 1972; Kimmel, 1974; Maris, 1969a, 1969b; M. Miller, 1978; Sendbuehler & Goldstein, 1977). White males over 65 have a suicide rate four times the national average; whereas white females over 65 have a rate twice the national average (Resnik & Cantor, 1970; Sendbuehler & Goldstein, 1977). In the United States, white males 65 and over commit suicide three times more often than white males aged 20–24 (Resnik & Cantor, 1970). Sainsbury (1968) found a similar trend in England, where the rate for males aged 60 and over was five times higher than the rate for males under 40. In 1978, the elderly male suicide rate in this country was 26.5 per 100,000, a dramatically high rate relative to the suicide rate for the United States as a whole, which has remained between 9 and 13 per 100,000 since World War II (M. Miller, 1978; U.S. Bureau of the Census, 1980).

The elderly white male suicide rate is significantly higher than the elderly white female rate. Overall the ratio is roughly 3:1 (Niccolini, 1973). The suicide rate for white females reaches a peak in mid-life and then declines, whereas the male suicide rate continues to increase through the eighth decade of life (Breed & Huffine, 1979; Bromley, 1966; Kaplan, 1979; M. Miller, 1979; Sainsbury, 1962). The ratio of male to female suicides in the 65–69 age group is about 4:1, but by age 85 the ratio is about 12:1 (Kastenbaum & Aisenberg, 1972; M. Miller, 1979; Rachlis, 1970; Weiss, 1968). This disparity in rates has also been found for almost all European countries except Norway and Finland (Atchley, 1980; Dublin, 1963; Kastenbaum & Aisenberg, 1972; Sainsbury, 1968). Table 1 graphically illustrates the suicide rate in the United States in 1978 by age and sex.

An interesting change in elderly male suicide rates has occurred since 1950. The suicide rate for white males aged 65–74 has declined 26 percent since 1950 (Resnik & Cantor, 1970). Marshall (1978) notes that the suicide rate for white males aged 65–74 in 1972 was less than 60 percent of the 1947 rate; whereas the rate for elderly white females remained about the same from 1947 to 1972. McIntosh and Santos (1981) noted similar declines in suicide rates for elderly white males, as well as elderly nonwhite males.

Race

Elderly suicide rates for nonwhites are considerably lower than for whites (Busse & Pfeiffer, 1969; McIntosh & Santos, 1981; M. Miller, 1979; Niccolini, 1973). The ratio of elderly white to elderly nonwhite suicides in the later age groups is approximately 3:1 (Niccolini, 1973). In 1982, the suicide rate for all white males was 20.0. The suicide rate for white males 65 and over was 39.2. The suicide rate for all black males in 1982 was 11.6. The rate for black males 65 and over was 12.9 (U.S. Bureau of the Census, 1982).

The trend for whites is an increase in suicides through the last stages of the life cycle. By contrast, minority suicide rates peak between 25–30 years of age and then decline through the later stages of the life cycle (McIntosh & Santos, 1981; Resnik & Cantor, 1970). Resnik and Cantor (1970) found suicide rates for blacks and whites to be roughly equal until age 35, when the rate for

Table 1 United States Suicide by Age and Sex, 1978

5-Year Age Group	Suicide Rates	
	Male	Female
5–9	0.0	0.0
10–14	1.2	0.4
15–19	12.8	3.1
20–24	27.4	6.4
25–29	27.5	7.9
30–34	23.4	8.3
35–39	22.3	9.3
40–44	21.4	11.0
45–49	22.5	11.1
50–54	24.3	11.3
55–59	25.4	10.8
60–64	30.1	8.4
65–69	30.2	8.3
70–74	37.2	7.4
75–79	45.9	8.4
80–84	50.6	6.0
85+	48.3	5.1

Source: Elderly Suicide Data Bases: Levels, Availability, Omission (p. 19) by J. L. McIntosh. Paper presented at the Annual Meeting of the Gerontological Society of America, San Francisco, California, November 1983. Reprinted with permission.

whites becomes two to three times higher. Table 2 vividly displays differences in suicide rates by age and race in the United States in 1978.

There is a great diversity among racial groups incorporated in the nonwhite category (Breed & Huffine, 1979; McIntosh & Santos, 1981). For instance, suicide rates of Chinese-Americans are higher than those of whites at all ages; however, those of American Indians are higher only in youth (Kramer, Pollack, Redick, & Locke, 1972). Data on specific minority groups are sparse; however, available data suggest that each group displays its own characteristic age pattern of suicide (McIntosh & Santos, 1981). McIntosh & Santos (1981) found that suicide rates are highest among the old for Chinese-Japanese and Filipino-Americans. By contrast, suicide among elderly blacks and native Americans is rare. These data are presented in Table 3.

Marital Status

As early as 1897, Emile Durkheim reported that suicide varied by age, gender, and marital status. Most notable in the data he assembled was the

Table 2 United States Suicide by Age and Sex, 1978

5-Year Age Group	Suicide Rates White	Suicide Rates Nonwhite
5–9	0.0	0.0
10–14	0.9	0.5
15–19	8.7	4.5
20–24	17.5	13.8
25–29	17.9	15.4
30–34	16.2	12.2
35–39	16.2	11.9
40–44	17.2	8.4
45–49	17.8	8.7
50–54	18.7	8.4
55–59	19.1	6.4
60–64	19.7	7.6
65–69	19.4	6.2
70–74	21.1	7.5
75–79	24.3	8.8
80–84	23.2	6.9
85+	20.0	6.3

Source: Elderly Suicide Data Bases: Levels, Availability, Omission (p. 21) by J. L. McIntosh. Paper presented at the Annual Meeting of the Gerontological Society of America, San Francisco, California, November 1983. Reprinted with permission.

markedly high ratio of suicides of men: three to every woman. His classic explanation for the greater proportion of suicides among widowers as compared to widows, namely, that men derive more from marriage than women, reflects this important gender difference among those growing older (Durkheim, 1897/1951).

Nonmarried persons at all ages are more likely to commit suicide than are married persons (Breed & Huffine, 1979; Durkheim, 1897/1951; Kastenbaum & Aisenberg, 1972). Studies have consistently revealed that the elderly who have lost spouses are particularly vulnerable to committing suicide (Gubrium, 1974; Kopell, 1977; MacMahon & Pugh, 1965; Maris, 1969a, 1969b; M. Miller, 1978; Payne, 1975; Resnik & Cantor, 1970). In particular, elderly widowers represent the most "at-risk" group for suicide (Berardo, 1967, 1968, 1970; Bock & Webber, 1972; Townsend, 1968).

Table 3 Suicide and Suicide Rates, U.S. Racial Minorities, 1976

Group	Age	Suicides	Rate	% Suicides	% Population
White	Total	24,854	13.35	100.00	100.00
	65+	4,380	21.02	17.62	11.19
	85+	351	19.71	1.41	0.96
Nonwhite	Total	1,978	6.95	100.00	100.00
	65+	169	8.02	8.54	7.40
	85+	20	10.64	1.01	0.66
Black	Total	1,614	6.52	100.00	100.00
	65+	134	7.14	8.30	7.58
	85+	15[a]	9.09	0.93	0.67
Indian	Total	175	19.16	100.00	100.00
	65+	2[a]	3.45	1.14	6.35
	85+	0	...	...	0.70
Chinese	Total	55	9.09	100.00	100.00
	65+	10[a]	23.07	18.18	7.16
	85+	0	...	...	0.52
Japanese	Total	56	8.59	100.00	100.00
	65+	13	22.51	23.21	8.86
	85+	5[a]	68.13	8.93	1.13
Filipino	Total	20	3.38	100.00	100.00
	65+	6[a]	13.26	30.00	7.65
	85+	0	...	...	0.39

[a]Rates based on very small numbers; thus they are subject to extreme fluctuation and should be viewed with caution.

Source: "Suicide among minority elderly: A preliminary investigation" by J. L. McIntosh and J. F. Santos, 1981, *Suicide and Life-Threatening Behavior, 11,* p. 155. Copyright 1981 by Human Sciences Press, Inc. Reprinted with permission.

Social Class and Occupation

In his classic study *Le Suicide: Étude de Sociologie,* Durkheim (1897/1951) described suicide as mainly an upper class phenomenon, suggesting that, unlike their fellows in lower socioeconomic classes, members of the upper class have fewer external restraints and controls on their behavior, resulting in higher rates of suicide. Since Durkheim's original work, a body of literature on the relationship between social class and suicide has developed. Although some studies have found suicide most prevalent among members of the upper class, most of the studies have revealed higher rates of suicide for members of the lower socioeconomic classes, including elderly members of the lower classes (Bock & Webber, 1972; Breed, 1963; Gardner, Bahn, & Mack, 1964; Maris, 1967, 1969a; Sainsbury, 1963; Stengel, 1964; Weiss, 1968).

Occupation has been used as a major indicator of social class position in the United States. Most studies confirm that suicide rates are highest among those in low-status occupations (Dublin, 1963; Dublin & Bunzel, 1933; Maris, 1967; Powell, 1958; Sainsbury, 1968).

Research studies have also confirmed a direct relationship between suicide and downward social mobility, occasioned by job loss or "occupational skidding" (Batchelor, 1957; Breed, 1963; Gardner et al., 1964; Maris, 1967, 1969a). Retirement in our society may be viewed as mandatory, culturally imposed, age-specific occupational skidding. Numerous researchers have implied a relationship between retirement and suicide (Batchelor, 1957; Breed & Huffine, 1979; Butler, 1975; Farberow & Moriwaki, 1975; Kopell, 1977; M. Miller, 1976, 1979; Sainsbury, 1962, 1968; Wolff, 1971).

Living Environment

Environment has a major effect on human behavior. Suicide rates are highest for those elderly living in urban areas, particularly in lower class, inner-city neighborhoods experiencing social disorganization (Cavan, 1928; Gardner et al., 1964; Henry & Short, 1954; Sainsbury, 1963; Schmid, 1928).

Another important predictor of suicide in the aged is isolation, desolation, or loneliness. The negative effect of social isolation has been identified as a key variable in elderly suicides (Gubrium, 1974; Sainsbury, 1963; Shanas et al., 1968; Townsend, 1968; Tunstall, 1966). In his study of suicides in London, Sainsbury (1955) found the percentage of suicides living alone was as high as 29.7 percent for all ages and was 39 percent for those aged 60 and over. In a more recent study of suicides among the elderly, Lonnqvist (1977) found that 33 percent of the male suicides were living alone, the corresponding percentage in the normal population being only 19 percent. Barraclough (1971) found that nearly half of the elderly suicides he studied were permanently living alone, whereas only 20 percent of the older population lived in one-person households. Maris (1969) similarly found that male suicides tended to live alone in attics or in skid-row hotels or apartments and were physically and socially isolated. Elderly male widowers are particularly isolated geographically, socially, and emotionally and, as a result, are even more vulnerable to suicide (Berardo, 1970; Bock, 1972; Bock & Webber, 1972; Maris, 1969a).

Two other factors have been related to elderly suicide: moving, and fear of institutionalization and dependency. In his analysis of factors precipitating suicide, Sainsbury (1973) found that suicides had moved significantly more often than controls. Analyses by age further revealed that elderly men are the most vulnerable to effects of moving. M. Miller (1979) found that fear of being institutionalized and then becoming dependent was a major precipitating factor in elderly suicide.*

THEORETICAL EXPLANATIONS AND CONCEPTUAL MODELS

Many explanations—drawn from sociology, psychology, and other disciplines—have been offered to explain the significantly higher rate of suicide among the old, as compared to other age groups, and to explain why particular groups of elderly are more vulnerable than others. In this section, a broad overview of these perspectives is presented. The section concludes with an attempt to integrate these various perspectives into a hypothetical predictive model of elderly suicide.

The Cultural Context

When Durkheim (1933/1964) suggested that "suicide is the ransom price of civilization" he was referring to the fact that in more urbanized, modernized, technologically developed countries the suicide rate is higher. Durkheim attributed the higher suicide rate in more modern societies to increased individuation of members, division of labor and specialization of tasks, and complexity. Most of the early nineteenth century investigators of suicide attributed the general rise in suicide rates to the dissolution of traditional social order and the transition to industrial civilization with its concomitants of "rationality" and individualism. Falret (1822) proposed that suicide was the result of both "internal causes" and "external causes," such as rapid social change. Many writers before Durkheim had already documented that suicide is more frequent in urban areas, in periods of great social change, and in economic depression. Morselli (1882/1979) had suggested that urbanization, civilization, and social complexity are conducive to suicide.

Modernized countries have a higher suicide rate than underdeveloped countries. Quinney (1965), in a study of 48 countries, found that in countries where urbanization or industrialization was increasing faster, the suicide rate was higher. Lynn (1969) carried out a cross-cultural study of suicide in Western countries and also found a significant positive correlation between economic growth and the suicide rate. These countries also had a large number of older individuals who comprised a large percentage of the population, a phenomenon referred to by demographers as a "maturing" of the population. It has been demonstrated that countries whose populations have a longer life expectancy have a higher suicide rate than countries whose populations have a shorter life expectancy. It is possible that the suicide rate is higher in more developed, modernized societies because of the larger number of older members, who more frequently kill themselves, thus pushing the suicide rate up for such countries. Demographic factors may be important if the aged are numerous and the role structure of the society fails to absorb the population. Mizruchi (1982) suggests that a numerical surplus population segment can become superfluous and therefore structurally disadvantaged if opportunities to participate in society are absent and people are held in terminal rather than transitional positions. Support for this notion comes from Atchley's (1980) study of suicide in various societies. Atchley found that societies that have high chronic disease rates also have high suicide rates, especially among those 65 and over. Studies conducted in Hong Kong and West Berlin have revealed increased suicide rates in those cities, both of which have experienced demographic changes in age composition as a result of immigration and emigration (Stengel & Cook, 1961).

Societies that place a high value on age have low suicide rates in their older populations. When societies modernize and industrialize, the rates of elderly self-destruction increase. As Seiden (1983) recently noted, "As cultures become less traditional, when age is no longer seen as a pathway to wisdom, when extended families fly to the wind, when people are considered interchangeable parts, when progress is highly valued, the suicide rates of the elderly will rise" (p. 5).

Cowgill and Holmes (1972) developed a cross-societal theory of aging, demonstrating a strong relationship between level of modernization in society (based on level of technology, degree of urbanization, rate of social change, and degree of westernization) and status of the aged. They concluded that, in Western, technologically advanced societies, the aged are devalued and hold less power, status, and economic control than in less advanced, more "backward" societies. Their theory gained support from Palmore and Manton's (1974) cross-cultural study in 31 countries, which demonstrated that the status of the aged is lower in more modernized countries. Suicide rates of the aged are highest in urban, industrialized countries, such as the United States (Quinney, 1965).

Rosow (1967) argues that the relative position of the aged in any society is governed by six institutional factors: (1) their ownership of property and control over the opportunities of the young, (2) their command of strategic knowledge and skills, (3) strong religiosity and sacred traditions, (4) strong kinship and extended family bonds in a communal or "Gemeinschaft" type of social organization, (5) a low-productivity economy, and (6) high mutual dependence and reciprocal aid among members. In American society, according to Rosow, the aged suffer a loss of status position on all these institutional dimensions.

American society highly values youth and beauty, productivity, progress, speed, and independence. In his classic study of American society, Williams (1970) concluded that occupational success is not just one life goal among others in American society, but is rather *the* outstanding trait of American culture. Mizruchi's (1964) work further confirms the emphasis on work and success in our society. Retired from participation in occupational roles, the elderly may suffer a severe loss of status, role, and power, as well as a loss of income, in our society.

The elderly in this country are often viewed as useless, dependent, nonproductive—a burden to be borne by younger members of the society. The elderly are "over the hill, down the drain, out to pasture, fading fast" (Butler, 1975, p. 2). They are often the victims of ageism and/or negative stereotyping. Images of aging in books, cartoons, well-known jokes and sayings and in the media present a picture of the elderly as sexless and senile, grumpy and cranky, wrinkled and toothless, and rigid and conservative in their values and thinking. As Troll, J. Israel, and K. Israel (1977) suggest, the stereotype of the elderly woman in this country portrays her as "poor, dumb, and ugly" (p. 4). The elderly in this country are advised to buy cremes to cover up "those ugly age spots and wrinkles," to join health and figure spas and try all sorts of diets to "keep that youthful figure." Hair dyes to "get rid of that ugly gray," dentures and tooth polish to "recapture that youthful smile," and tonics and pills to "feel young and look young again" are also available. If all of these remedies fail to transform an old face and figure into a young one, the multibillion dollar cosmetic business in the United States surely can perform the miracle.

Thus, in our youth-oriented, production-minded society, the aged are devalued. Their skills become obsolete in the face of rapid technological change. Their wisdom and experience, gained from years of living, are not valued by many in the younger generations who confront a different world from the one in which their parents and grandparents lived.

How do the elderly view themselves in such a culture? Presumably, when all of the diets and pills and cremes and cosmetics fail, the elderly are forced to see themselves as old. Indeed, many accept the negative cultural images and, consequently, their self-esteem and self-concept suffer.

The Sociological Perspective

Although earlier writers had reported a relationship between suicide rates and various variables, the first well-known sociological study of suicide was conducted in 1897 by Emile Durkheim. Durkheim's *Suicide* (1897/1951) has exerted a major influence on sociology as a discipline and served as a blueprint for later sociological studies of suicide in particular. In his work, Durkheim, influenced by the earlier work of Morselli (1882/1979) and others, attempted to demonstrate that suicide cannot be explained by psychological or biological factors alone. Durkheim held that the nature and extent of one's involvement in society is a decisive factor in suicide and that various social factors, over which the individual has little or no control, are important in understanding the variations in suicide rates.

> First of all, it can be said that, as collective force is one of the obstacles best calculated to restrain suicide, its weakening involves a development of suicide. When society is strongly integrated, it holds individuals under its control, considers them at its service and thus forbids them to dispose willfully of themselves.... There is, in short, in a cohesive and animated society, a constant interchange of ideas and feelings from all to each and each to all, something like a mutual moral support, which instead of throwing the individual on his own resources, leads him to share in the collective energy and supports his own when exhausted. (Durkheim, 1897/1951, pp. 209–210)

In other words, the nature and extent of one's involvement in society is an important determining influence on one's vulnerability to suicide.

Durkheim sought explanations for variations in the suicide rate in terms of the degree to which people are integrated in the society and the extent to which their conduct is regulated (Giddens, 1971). He derived two major propositions: (1) that the suicide rate varies inversely with the degree of integration of the group, and (2) that the suicide rate varies inversely with the degree of normative regulation.

Regarding the former, suicide varies with the strength of bonds between the person and the groups with which the person is affiliated. Thus, not only are persons more vulnerable to suicide if they are too weakly integrated into groups, which provide meaning and control over their lives, but excessive integration also increases their proclivity to suicide.

What Durkheim called integration has something to do with a person's social ties to the larger group, with a person's level of meaningful interaction with other members of the larger social group, with that person's degree of social "belongingness."

> A society, group, or social condition is said to be integrated to the degree that its members possess a "common conscience" of shared beliefs and sentiments, interact with one another and have a sense of devotion to common goals. In a condition of weak integration, life derives no meaning and purpose from the group (Johnson, 1965, p. 876).

Durkheim suggested that happiness depends on one finding a sense of meaning outside oneself, which occurs only in the context of group involvement. One of the major elements of integration is the extent to which various members of a society interact with one another. Related to the frequency of patterned interaction is a measure of value integration, "the sharing by members of values and beliefs" (Durkheim, 1964).

In his famous typology of suicide, Durkheim describes two types resulting from man's level of integration into society. He postulated that persons who are deeply and intimately involved with others in various social groups should be low suicide risks. He consequently found the unmarried to have the highest rate of suicide. He identified the type of suicide that results from lack of integration as "egoistic." According to Durkheim, the stronger the forces throwing one onto one's own resources, the greater the likelihood of egoistic suicide. Durkheim classified suicide among the aged as "egoistic." He proposed that suicide increases with age because society as a moral force begins to recede from the person, in terms of both goals and commitments, as the person ages and withdraws from various roles and positions. The older individual is less integrated into and less dependent upon society.

Building on the early work of Durkheim, Rosow (1967) suggested that the elderly tend to be less integrated into society due to (1) their removal and withdrawal from certain organizational contexts and associated roles, thereby weakening their ties to mediating structures, such as work, voluntary associations, and like organizations; and (2) the contraction of their intimate social world, which results from relocation, incapacitation, and death of friends and peers. In comparison to other age groups, the elderly belong to fewer formal and informal social groups (Babchuck & Booth, 1969; Booth, 1972; Dotson, 1951) and also have fewer friendships (Blau, 1973; Rosow, 1967).

According to Rosow (1973), the integration of the elderly into society is seriously weakened as a result of the loss of major social roles in the family, the world of work, and society in general.

First, the loss of roles excludes the aged from significant social participation and devalues them. It deprives them of vital functions that underlie their sense of worth, their self-conceptions and their self-esteem. In a word, they are depreciated and become marginal, alienated from the larger society. (Rosow, 1973, p. 82)

Not only are the elderly more likely to commit "egoistic suicide" because of their lack of integration into formal and informal social groups, they are also more likely to commit "anomic suicide." As Rosow (1973) and Neugarten (1968) point out, our culture does not provide older members with definitions and meaningful norms, so older persons are left to structure the "aged role" for themselves, with no clear prescriptions as to the appropriate behavior. Durkheim refers to this condition as "anomie."

Old age, unlike other stages in the life cycle, is also the first stage of life with systematic status loss, as Rosow (1973) aptly points out. All other statuses, from childhood through adolescence to full maturity, are normally marked by steady social acquisitions of power, prestige, and rewards. When people enter the later stages of life and assume the aged role, however, for the first time loss of status is experienced. They now realize that the life goals they set for themselves may never be attained, as the resources for achieving them dwindle before their eyes.

Another factor producing a greater probability of suicide in the elderly results from the changes in expectations associated with stages in the life cycle. Norms of achievement, which operated throughout the earlier stages, now give way to relatively amorphous norms of ascription as the bases of judging the behavior of the elderly. Persons pass into a stage in which they become socially defined as old, in which the basis of judgment shifts from criteria of performance to those of age, regardless of accomplishment (Rosow, 1973).

In sum, older age status appears to be accompanied by decreasing opportunity to function as an effective member of the society and by an increasing inability to achieve life goals. This pattern may be expected to result in despair, demoralization, and uneasiness.

In his book, Durkheim reported that suicide varied by age and gender. Most notable was the markedly high ratio, 3:1, of suicides of men compared to that of women. His classic explanation for the greater proportion of suicides among widowers, as compared to widows, was that men derive more from marriage than women (Durkheim, 1897/1951).

Durkheim recognized that participation in the family represented one of the most important ties among society's members. He suggested that the state of marriage and membership in a family integrate societal members by exerting a regulative force on them and by acting as a stimulant to intensive interpersonal relations that draw the members into firm and meaningful union, thus providing some degree of immunity, the "coefficient of preservation," against suicide. Durkheim explained higher rates of suicide among widows and widowers as due to "domestic anomie," that is, a deregulation of behavior resulting from the spouse's death. He also viewed the loss of the spouse as weakening the familial integration of the individual. Thus, the suicide of widows and widowers may be referred to as both "anomic" and "egoistic." Berardo (1968, 1970) similarly describes the situation of widows and widowers as vague and unstructured, lacking clear guidelines for behavior, and lacking supportive interaction with friends, kin, and coworkers. Two other followers of Durkheim, Henry and Short (1954), have explained suicide in terms of the weakening of the relational system constituted by marriage; and Bock (1972) points out that "marriage not only integrates the individual into a close and meaningful association but also regulates him by requiring him to take the other person into account in activities and decisions" (p. 72).

The elderly widower is likely to be the most socially isolated and the most vulnerable to suicide (Berardo, 1967, 1968, 1970; Bock, 1972; Bock & Webber, 1972; Gubrium, 1974; Maris, 1969a). He has fewer relatives and kin living nearby, participates less with family and friends, and is less involved in formal organizations and the community. As Berardo points out, the situation of both widows and widowers is difficult because of the lack of clear-cut expectations, but this is felt more acutely by the widower who, unlike the widow, is unfamiliar with domestic and other roles not associated with a formal occupation. Coupled with this is the fact that females have traditionally maintained kin and friend networks.

Durkheim considered the occupational group, endowed with political status, to be particularly cohesive and to constitute the richest channel for a common life. He advocated reintegration in modern industrial society through intermediate occupational groups. Powell (1970) notes that the male is primarily integrated into American society through the occupational role. If one accepts Powell's assumption that occupation constitutes a basis of status integration for members of American society, particularly men, then one must conclude that the absence or deprivation of occupation results in loss of status integration or loss of status. Accordingly, many retired men may be viewed as living in a condition of anomie.

Aged white males in America suffer the most severe status loss of any group. Maris (1969a), Breed (1963), and Powell (1970) have all related the high suicide rates of elderly white males to the severe loss of status, power, money, and role relationships formerly provided by participation in work. By comparison, women generally and minority males, two groups that traditionally have held lower status positions in our society, have less to lose upon retirement than white males and thus tend to display lower rates of suicide than white males in our society. Maris (1969a) and Seiden (1981) both attribute the lower rate of suicide among older blacks, as compared to older whites, to the greater degree of external constraint imposed upon blacks and to their more intense involvement in family, church, and other social relational systems. Seiden (1981) argues that elderly blacks are wanted and needed in the family system, sometimes due to economic necessity, but also because old age is respected by blacks, and they therefore feel they belong and are useful and productive. According to Seiden, the intense support networks and strong human relationships that characterize the black community protect elderly blacks against suicide.

A related sociological position, derived from the symbolic interactionist's perspective, is role theory (Blau, 1973; Lopata, 1973). Symbolic interactionists posit that individuals derive an identity and sense of self through interaction with significant others in the performance of social roles in groups. Some sources of identity are more important than others, that is, some relationships, such as marriage, are more likely to involve "significant others." According to Hughes (1981), some roles are associated with "master status" and have a greater impact on the self and on one's identity than others. The occupational role is a "master status" in our society, particularly for males.

Loss of social roles, according to this perspective, results in a loss of identity and subsequent loss of esteem, lowered self-concept, and a sense of meaninglessness in life. From this perspective, the loss of a spouse and retirement are viewed as major losses of social roles, placing the individual outside the normal group of patterned associations—associations that formerly served to locate the individual in a matrix of other roles and provide a sense of identity and meaning.

The identity crisis theory of retirement (S. J. Miller, 1965; Phillips, 1957) argues that work is the major, culturally dominant role for males in our society and the major source of social status, self-respect, and identity. According to this position, leisure roles and other nonwork roles can not provide the retiree with adequate substitutes for the lost role of the worker. Therefore, retirement results in a major loss of self-respect and social status, lowered self-concept and morale, and crisis of identity. The theory holds that retirement is a negative status, signifying that one is old, useless, and no longer a vital, contributing member of the community (Thompson, 1973).

S. J. Miller (1965) presents the most elaborate statement of the identity crisis theory. Writing on the crisis of retirement and its concomitant loss of identity, he states:

> The occupational identity is that which provides the social substance by which other identities are maintained, various roles are coordinated, and the appropriateness of social activity is substantiated. In other words, the retired person finds himself without a role which would justify his social future. (p. 72)

The symbolic interactionists hold that the self-image is formed by taking into account the perspective of "significant others." If a person has relied on another person to predict and act in many ways as an extension of one's self, then the loss of that person is tantamount to losing a part of one's self. Thus, the loss of a spouse changes the basis of self-identity, particularly for women (Lopata, 1973; Weigert & Hastings, 1977).

In our society, the nuclear family is not only the major provider of emotional support and haven from the troubles of a fast-paced, complex world, but also the major unit of recreation and association. When a spouse dies, in addition to losing the role of the husband or wife, the widowed individual also often loses friendship and associational roles. For many, an emotional void and overpowering loneliness often accompanies the loss of such an important role as spouse (Lopata, 1973).

Blau (1956) has offered an explanation for the dramatically higher rates of suicide among elderly males, reflecting the role theory perspective. In her work, Blau noted the negative effect of cumulative role loss: the more social roles lost, the greater the negative impact. Elderly males lose their roles in two major social institutions in society: work and the family. The male may have relied strongly on "his occupation and co-workers earlier in his life for social and personal identity, and retirement may have forced him to depend more heavily on his spouse for personal social significance. Under these conditions, her death would have meant even greater isolation from kin and community groups" (Blau, 1956, p. 62). Townsend (1968) has referred to this change or discontinuity in social engagements, experienced most acutely by male widowers who have lost roles in the work and family world, as "desolation."

Psychological Factors and Explanations

According to the classical theory of four humors, melancholy belongs to autumn and evening, and the threshold of old age is crossed at about age 60. Old age has been described as the season of losses. The losses suffered by the aged may be emotional (loss of spouse, child, or good friend), psychological (loss of self-esteem, self-confidence, or personal control and competence), physical (loss of hearing, sight, physical health, or mobility), social (loss of job or community activity), or financial (loss of status, power, and income).

Although he primarily emphasized social forces as causes of suicide, Durkheim recognized and noted the intimate connection between losses in the social realm and those in the psychological realm. In *Suicide* he notes that egoism is said to be accompanied by "collective currents of depression and disillusionment" and by "miserable weariness and sad depression" (Durkheim, 1897/1951, pp. 214, 225).

Freud is recognized as the father of psychological explanations of suicide. In his early work, Freud (1917/1955) contended that loss of a loved one results in feelings of abandonment and rejection, which may swell into anger directed against the lost loved one. Loss results in a particular state of mind in the individual. In an attempt to kill the memory of the lost loved one, suicide may result. In his later works, Freud (1920/1955) postulated the existence in each human being of a death instinct (Thanatos), which, in the case of suicidal intent, may overcome the life instinct (Eros).

One of Freud's main contributions to suicidology derives from his clinical studies of depressed patients. Freud (1917/1955) stated that the self-hatred seen in depression originates in anger toward a love object that is turned back on the self, the idea of "retroflexed rage" or "murder in the 180th degree." The underlying assumption in Freud's work is that a person commits suicide because the person originally intended to kill someone else. This idea was earlier enunciated by Stekel (1918), who claimed that "no one kills himself who has not wished to kill another" (p. 338).

Freud's concept of suicide was psychoanalytical. For Freud, suicide was essentially a result of mental processes associated with depression. Suicide, in other words, was an intrapsychic process and represented unconscious hostility directed toward an introjected, ambivalently viewed love object. One killed one's self to murder the hurtful image or memory of one's love-hated father (mother, friend, etc.) within one's own self.

According to Freud, all depressed individuals are potential suicides. The distinguishing features of melancholia, according to Freud (1917), are profoundly painful dejection, loss of interest in the outside world, inability to love, inhibition of all activity, and feelings of reproach and self-condemnation. Unlike the person suffering from normal grief, melancholic persons picture themselves as worthless and morally despicable; but they are, at the same time, overbearing and make unrealistic demands on those around them.

Influenced by Freud's earlier work, several psychological explanations of suicide have focused on the concepts of loss and depression as they affect the state of mind of the individual and perhaps induce suicide. Loss plays a role in bringing about depression and in determining its course and severity. According to M. Miller (1979), when several major losses occur in close temporal proximity and when the resistance of the individual is low, the likelihood of suicide is greatest.

The loss of a love object (narcissistic supply) has been identified as of major significance in the etiology of depression and suicide. Since Freud's classical work, *Mourning and Melancholia* (1917), in which he noted the close similarities between melancholia and normal grief suffered upon the loss of a loved object, Parkes (1965), Glick, Weiss, and Parkes (1974), Bornstein, Clayton, Halikas, Maurice, and Rogins (1973), and others have similarly identified depression as a major feature of the normal grief process. Winokur (1974) has called bereavement the "paradigm of reactive depression."

Based on his indepth study of victims who lost "significant others" in the Cocoanut Grove fire, Lindemann (1944) identified the following symptoms associated with normal grief: somatic distress (fatigue, feelings of tightness in the throat, pains in the stomach and chest, changes in sleeping and eating patterns), preoccupation with the image of the deceased, guilt, restlessness and anxiety, hostility, and changed patterns of social activity and conduct (withdrawing from clubs, activities, and friendship circles). Since Lindemann first noted these symptoms of normal grief, many of which are also characteristic of reactive depression, other students of grief have confirmed Lindemann's findings (Caine, 1974; Clayton, Halikas, & Maurice, 1971; Lopata, 1973; MacMahon & Pugh, 1965; Vachon, 1976).

Individuals who have lost their spouses are sad and lonely. When their spouses are gone they often feel parts of themselves have died. Life becomes empty and meaningless when their most significant persons—those who have laughed with them and cried with them, shared special moments and secrets with them, and always been there when they needed them—are gone. They are often filled with fear and anxiety when their two-person world is suddenly turned upside down and they must face life alone. They are overcome with anguish and despair, for they can not imagine that anything or anyone can ever take the place of that which has been lost. In Goethe's words:

> Numbed, distracted, she finds herself at the edge of a precipice. Naught but shadows surround her. No perspective, no consolation, no presentiment. For the only one who made her feel alive has left her. She does not see at all how vast is the world, or the many others in it who could replace what she has lost. She feels herself one, abandoned by all. The future closes up again before her. (Halbwachs, 1930, p. 271)

MacMahon and Pugh (1965) and M. Miller (1979) have noted that the first year after bereavement is the greatest time of risk for suicide.

It is no wonder that the elderly, confronted as they are with multiple stresses and losses, suffer more from depression than younger individuals. Research data reveal that 15 percent of all persons aged 65 and over are depressed (Lauter, 1973). For those in poor health, the proportion of depressives may be as high as 50 percent (Dovenmuehle & Verwoerdt, 1962). Depression is the most common functional psychiatric disorder of late life (Pfeiffer, 1977; Salzman and Shader, 1979).

Kastenbaum (1964) discusses old age not only as an unexpected event but also as a profound misfortune in which individuals are faced with the difficult task of explaining to themselves and others how it came to pass that they are not what they used to be. Such individuals experience what Kastenbaum refers to as the "crisis of explanation." For these persons, growing old brings a very negative self-evaluation and loss of self-esteem; they can not accept or explain the new old self and, therefore, they lose their earlier identity.

Self-hatred and low self-esteem are at the root of suicidal behavior. When the discrepancy between performance and ambition is very great, as is often the case in late life, the resultant carrot-and-stick situation further hastens negative changes in self-concept. Changes in appearance that accompany the aging process (wrinkled skin, graying hair, memory loss, slowed reaction time, easy fatigability, loss of stamina, uncertainty of gait, greater vulnerability to infections and chronic illnesses, and reduced keenness of all five senses) negatively affect the person's self-image. The overemphasis on youth and beauty in our culture further contributes to the negative self-concept and lowered self-esteem of the aged.

Bibring (1953) developed the theory that depression is an ego state in which the feeling of helplessness is the basic underlying dynamic. Seligman (1975, 1976) defines helplessness as a state in which individuals experience an inability to control or predict significant life events and suggests that it is the core of all depression. He notes that "the depressed patient believes or has learned that he cannot control those elements of his life that relieve suffering, bring gratification, or provide nurture—in short, he believes that he is helpless" (1975, p. 92). The aged are the most susceptible to helplessness, according to Seligman, because they have experienced the greatest loss of control. Schulz (1976) similarly argues that the loss of job, income, physical health, work, and child-rearing roles results in increased helplessness and depression in the aged. Appelbaum (1963) and Stengel (1964) have also identified the basic feelings of helplessness as a factor in suicide.

Followers of Freud have continued to view suicide as a result of unconscious mental processes, instincts, or drives. Menninger (1938) argued that suicide is largely the result of "unconscious psychological factors" rather than the result of social or personal disorganization, as Cavan and other sociologists had claimed. Menninger, like Freud, viewed suicide as an act of displaced murder, as "murder in the 180th degree" (p. 29). Every true suicidal act, according to Menninger, contains three elements: the wish to kill (sadism), the wish to be killed (masochism), and the wish to die (submission).

Thus, Menninger accepted Freud's concept of a death instinct (Thanatos). Menninger visualized suicide as the winning out of destructive tendencies over constructive ones under conditions of stress and conflict. In emphasizing the wish to die as the major motive in elderly suicide, Menninger identified hopelessness as a major contributing factor.

Influenced by Menninger's theory, Shneidman and Farberow (1957) analyzed the suicide notes from 610 completed suicides and found that the wish to die characterized 57 percent of the notes of older men and 75 percent of the notes left by elderly females; the notes of those aged 20–39 reflected only 23 percent and 21 percent, respectively, who wished to die. The elderly expressed feelings of discouragement, pain, and despair. Many said they were tired of living or of life.

Barraclough (1971) and Batchelor (1957) found that the elderly who are suicidal often talk of feeling tired of living or of dealing with the day-to-day problems or hassles of life. They experience a state of "psychological exhaustion." Kobler and Stotland (1964), who studied successful suicides, point directly to a loss of hope as the precipitating factor, noting that "suicide occurred in each case when, and only when, all significant hopeful relationships were broken" (p. 11).

Farber (1968) similarly conceived of suicide among the aged as a desperate response to hopeless, intolerable life situations: "Suicide occurs when there appears to be no available path that will lead to a tolerable existence . . . . It is when the life interest is one of despairing helplessness that suicide occurs" (p. 17). Farber defines hope as the relationship between a sense of personal competence and life-threatening events. When all hope of achieving life's goals or fulfilling life's dreams is gone, personal despair results.

Kierkegard (1849/1941) referred to despair as a "sickness unto death." Similarly, M. Miller (1979) has described the crossing of what he calls the "line of unbearability" as the major factor in elderly suicide:

> Lying dormant within all of us is an extremely personal equation which determines the point where the quality of our lives would be so pathetically poor we would no longer wish to live. This "line of unbearability," as it might be called, usually exists only subconsciously and we are therefore not normally cognizant of it. However, when we actually find ourselves in an intolerable situation, even for the first time in our lives, we become conscious of our "line of unbearability." Once the line of unbearability is crossed, a crisis is triggered. Those who still maintain hope cry out for help. Those who don't are likely to kill themselves quickly and with determination. (p. 8)

The psychological state that characterizes the suicide-prone is a state of intolerable despair—what Herman Melville refers to in *Moby Dick* (1964), a masterpiece of self-destruction, as "insufferable anguish". Individuals who see no tolerable path to a meaningful existence, who feel totally hopeless to better their lives or change their environment now or in the future, are the ones most likely to choose suicide when they encounter life's problems and frustrations.

PHYSICAL ILLNESS AND STRESS

The Illness Factor

Percy W. Bridgman, the Nobel Laureate in physics and a famous American philosopher, committed suicide August 20, 1961, at the age of 80. His suicide note, published in 1962 in the *Bulletin of the Atomic Scientist*, states, "It isn't decent for society to make man do this thing himself. Probably this is the last day I will be able to do it myself." Bridgman had cancer and was in great pain, and doctors had refused to give him a substance he had asked for to end his life.

The importance of physical illness as a factor in suicide among the elderly has been noted by several observers. Dorpat, Anderson, and Ripley (1968) found that, of the 60 completed suicides they studied, 70 percent of the subjects suffered from some illness. In those aged 60 and over, physical illness was the most common precipitating factor in suicide. Batchelor and Napier (1953) similarly observed in their study that 60 percent of the completed suicides of people aged 60 and over suffered from a physical ailment. M. Miller (1976) found that 62 percent of the suicides of elderly white males he studied were the result of physical illness. Maris (1969), Resnik and Cantor (1970), Gardner et al. (1964), Kay and Walk (1971), Murphy and Robins (1967), Benson and Brodie (1975), and Farberow and Moriwaki (1975) have also noted the relationship between physical illness and suicide in late life.

The aged, more than younger persons, suffer from painful, chronic, debilitating diseases, such as cancer, Parkinson's disease, arthritis, heart disease, and stroke. Among the many consequences of such diseases are pain and suffering, body disfigurement, anxiety, worry, depression, loss of self-esteem and self-confidence, interruption of significant life activities, and altered interpersonal relationships with "significant others." Illness places great physical stress on the aged body, which, due to physiological changes accompanying the aging process, is less able to endure such stress. Based on their reviews of several studies, Cohen and Lazarus (1979) suggest that illness poses threats to life, threats to bodily comfort and integrity, threats to self-concept and future plans, threats to one's emotional equilibrium, and threats to the fulfillment of customary social roles and activities in work, the family, and the community.

Illness may cause brooding and introspection and eventually result in the realization of one's frailty or of the threat of permanent dependency. The older person may have great difficulty evolving new values and a self-image that can tolerate and incorporate infirmity. Latent fears and anxieties about death grow real with illness. Pride in one's body and its resiliency is severely shaken in the face of a disease such as cancer. Indeed, Dubovsky (1978) has pointed out that self-destruction in cancer patients reflects the frustration and helplessness they experience when recovery is not forthcoming.

The Stress Model

Selye (1956) and others defined stress as the physical stimuli and emotional factors that place a strain on the homeostatic system. Stress is present when the defensive reactions of the organism are called into action. Stress has since been defined by Lazarus (1966) as the degree of imbalance between the demands of a life event or group of life events placed on a person and that person's ability to cope with the demands. Similarly, Holmes and Rahe (1967) have defined stress from a life events perspective. Their 42-item checklist of stressful life events remains one of the most popular instruments used to measure "stress."

A stressor is defined in the literature as anything that implies or causes threat or trauma to the organism. Stressful stimuli are novel, intense, and unexpected stimuli (Appley & Trumbull, 1967). External stressors include such events as retirement, loss of a spouse, or relocation; internal stressors refer to changes in bodily or mental function or to disease within the organism.

According to Selye (1946, 1955, 1974, 1976), stressors disturb the equilibrium of the individual and produce what he termed the general adaptation syndrome. This syndrome has three states: (1) alarm reaction, physiologically preparing the body for flight or fight, thereby activating the release of the adrenal cortex or corticosteroids into the blood stream; (2) the stage of resistance, in which all of the body's defenses are called upon to react to exposure to stimuli; and (3) exhaustion, which results from prolonged exposure to harmful stimuli to which adaptation could no longer be maintained. Stress depletes the individual through wear and tear and accelerates the aging process. Prolonged exposure to stress puts the individual into a state of protracted emotion and physiological preparation for flight or fight, which is often "blocked." Fatigue, eye twitching, and muscle pain are often the result of prolonged exposure to stress.

Stress has been demonstrated to have a negative effect on both physical health (B. S. Dohrenwend & B. P. Dohrenwend, 1974; Holmes & Rahe, 1967; Holmes & Masuda, 1974; Rabkin & Streuning, 1976) and mental health (Lowenthal & Haven, 1968; Payne, 1975) and to precipitate suicide (Paykel, Prusoff, & Myers, 1975). According to M. Miller (1979), "whether an older person is able to resolve a suicidal crisis or succumbs to self-inflicted death is very much a function of the ability to cope with stress" (p. 25). McIntosh, Hubbard, and Santos (1981), Rosow (1973), M. Miller (1979), and others have emphasized the importance of stress as a predictor of suicide among the elderly.

Loss—whether real, threatened, or imaginary—is a stress that requires readjustment to maintain equilibrium within the psychic structure. Late life represents a period of multiple stress at a time when the organism is least able to deal with it. Impaired ability to cope with stress has been noted as a major characteristic of the aging process by Eisdorfer and Wilkie (1977), Jarvik (1975), and Welford (1962). Failing health, chronic disease, impaired eyesight, hearing, and cognitive functioning, and weakened recuperative powers are all sources of stress in late life. Stress may also stem from loss of income, status, and power; loss of social roles in work, family, and the community; loss of family, friends and loved ones; loss of mobility and independence; loss of home and personal possessions; or isolation through physical disability. Rosow (1973) suggests that loss of social roles and function introduces stress because role loss excludes the aged from participation in work, family, and other social groups. Ageism and negative cultural images have also been noted as a source of stress in late life (Lehr, 1979; Loether, 1975; Payne, 1975). Blocked opportunity, or the discrepancy between life goals and the means of attaining them, has been identified as a cause of alienation, hopelessness, and powerlessness, and as a source of chronic stress for the aged.

The multiple stresses of aging require adaptation, flexibility, and resiliency if the individual is to survive, rather than succumb to suicide. Suicidal behavior among the elderly is often associated with the inability to cope with vital losses. M. Miller (1979) suggests that the factor that distinguishes those elderly who succumb to suicide when faced with multiple losses and stresses from those who supplant vital losses with new sources of satisfaction and survival is the ability to cope and the strength of the will to live.

Some older people are better suited than others to adjusting to the problems and losses experienced in late life. As Busse and Pfeiffer (1969) point out, "It has been customary to say that an individual's adaptation at any given point in time is determined by an interplay of the biological, psychological, social, and physiological factors impinging on him at that moment and in his recent and distant past" (p. 183). Bergman (1972) similarly concludes that genetic factors and early environmental experiences may be the most important factors in determining the ability of older persons to withstand stresses in late life.

M. Miller (1979) and McIntosh et al. (1981) point out that coping strategies that can be relied upon in late life are developed early in life and practiced and refined throughout adolescence and mid-life. In other words, how well one adapted to problems in young adulthood and mid-age is probably one of the best predictors of how well one will adapt to the problems and stresses of late life.

Seiden (1981) has explained the significantly low rates of nonwhite suicide in terms of lifetime adaptation, adjustment, and coping. Blacks who have lived with poverty and racism, as well as blocked educational and occupational opportunities, have learned to adjust their expectations and to cope with frustrations throughout life. As a result, the blows of aging affect them less than they do their white counterparts, who may have never had to learn to cope in younger years. Similarly, it is possible that women, who have always had to play a greater variety of roles than males and who have had to cope with more frustrations and blocked opportunities, commit suicide less frequently in late life because they too have learned earlier in life to be flexible and adaptable.

Other factors related to early life experiences and adjustments at other stages of the life cycle determine how well an elderly individual will adjust to the problems of late life. Busse and Pfeiffer (1969) note that:

> those who have developed trusting relationships with others, a clearly defined valued identity, a sense of autonomy, who have previously confronted adversity without succumbing to it, and who have performed satisfactorily in marriage and in work make the best adjustment in late life. (p. 184)

Good health, intelligence, involvement with close, intact families, educational opportunities, orderly careers, close friendships, and good marriages in younger years—all these factors will prepare one to adjust in late life.

In his study of suicides among the elderly, M. Miller (1979) found that a significantly greater percentage of people who had committed suicide had experienced either a broken home or been raised by domineering, critical, insensitive parents. In their study of 200 completed suicides, Batchelor and Napier (1953) discovered a history of broken homes in childhood in 50 percent of the elderly who had completed suicides and a family history of mental illness in 65 percent. Birren (1964) also found broken homes in childhood and a family history of mental illness as two major factors in geriatric suicide. Other studies have revealed that those elderly who commit suicide had personality characteristics like shyness, undue sensitivity, dependency, anxiety, and hypochondriasis that hampered the development of close interpersonal relationships throughout life (Batchelor & Napier, 1953; Maris, 1969; M. Miller, 1979).

Individuals who have previously used alcohol as a means to cope with life's problems are particularly "at risk" of suicide in late life (Barraclough, 1971; Gardner et al., 1964; M. Miller, 1979). Those who have attempted suicide earlier as a way to deal with the problems of daily living are also much more likely later to choose suicide as a solution (Batchelor, 1957; Kreitman, 1977; O'Neal, Robins, & Schmidt, 1956). Unsuccessful attempts in late life are more predictive of successful completion within one or two years after the attempt than are such attempts among the young.

CONCLUSIONS

Available statistics clearly demonstrate that the elderly are more prone to commit suicide than other age groups in the United States. Furthermore, certain groups of elderly are more at risk than others. Males, the unmarried, whites, those in lower socioeconomic classes and low-status occupations or who have experienced "occupational skidding," and the lonely and isolated in urban areas are the most susceptible to suicide.

Various explanations have been offered for the disproportionately higher rates of suicide among the aged, particularly white widowed males. Explanations have focused on multiple losses suffered by the elderly (physical, emotional, mental, financial, personal, and social) as they precipitate depression, clearly a causal factor in elderly suicide. The stress model identifies loss and depression as factors that impact on vulnerability to stress, ability to cope with stress, and suicide in the elderly. Finally, viewed in a larger cultural context, suicide is more characteristic of the aged in westernized, urbanized, industrialized societies than in preindustrialized or developing countries.

It is clear that there are many interrelated factors that predict suicide in the elderly. Indeed, as Barter (1969) has noted with respect to the etiology of elderly suicide, "A precipitating cause may be less obvious and the suicide may appear to be a reaction to a total life situation more than any single event" (p. 9).

Based on the various theories and findings we have examined, Figure 1 presents a hypothetical representation of the relationship between relevant factors in the aging process and suicide. The represented process is not an empirically established causal model, but it does suggest the types of relationships that should be examined more definitively in future research on the etiology of suicide in the elderly.

Figure 1 A Model of the Aging Process and Suicide

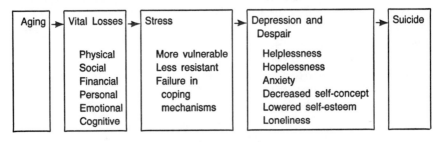

REFERENCES

Alvarez, A. (1972). *The savage god: A study of suicide.* New York: Random House.

Applebaum, S. A. (1963). The problem-solving aspect of suicide. *Journal of Projective Techniques, 27,* 259–268.

Appley, M. H., & Trumbull, R. (Eds.). (1967). *Psychological stress.* New York: Appleton-Century-Crofts.

Atchley, R. C. (1980). Aging and suicide: Reflections on the quality of life. In S. G. Haynes, M. Feinlib, J. A. Ross, & L. Stallones (Eds.), *Epidemiology of aging* (NIH Publication No. 8–969, pp. 141–161). Washington, D.C.: U.S. Department of Health and Human Services.

Babchuck, N., & Booth, A. (1969). Voluntary association membership: A longitudinal analysis. *American Sociological Review, 34,* 31–45.

Baqucher, J. (1979). *Suicide.* New York: Basic Books.

Barraclough, B. M. (1971). Suicide in the elderly. In D. W. Kay & A. Walk (Eds.), *Recent developments in psychogeriatrics* (pp. 89–97). Kent, England: Headly Brothers.

Barter, J. T. (1969). Self-destructive behavior in adolescents and adults: Similarities and differences. In U. S. Department of Health, Education & Welfare, *Suicide among the American Indians: Two workshops* (PHS Publication No. 1903, pp. 7–10). Washington, D.C.: U.S. Government Printing Office.

Batchelor, I. R. C. (1957). Suicide in old age. In E. S. Shneidman & N. L. Farberow (Eds.), *Clues to suicide* (pp. 143–151). New York, NY: McGraw-Hill.

Batchelor, I. R. C., & Napier, M. (1953). Attempted suicide in old age. *British Medical Journal, 2,* 1186–1190.

Benson, R., & Brodie, D. (1975). Suicide by overdoses of medicines among the aged. *Journal of the American Geriatrics Society, 23,* 304–308.

Berardo, F. M. (1967). Social adaptation to widowhood among a rural-urban aged population (Washington Agricultural Experiment Station Bulletin 689). Pullman, Wash.: Washington State University.

Berardo, F. M. (1968). Widowhood status in the U. S.: Perspectives on a neglected aspect of the family life cycle. *Family Coordinator, 17,* 191.

Berardo, F. M. (1970). Survivorship and social isolation: The case of the aged widower. *Family Coordinator, 19,* 11–25.

Bergman, K. (1972). Personality traits and reactions to the stresses of aging. In H. M. Van Praag & A. F. Kalverbor (Eds.), *Aging of the central nervous* system: *Biological and psychological aspects* (pp. 162–182). Haarlem, Netherlands: De Erven F. Bohn.

Bibring, E. (1953). The mechanism of depression. In P. Greenacre (Ed.), *Affective disorders* (pp. 13–48). New York: International Universities Press.

Birren, J. E. (1964). *The psychology of aging.* Englewood Cliffs, N.J.: Prentice-Hall.

Blau, Z. (1956). Changes in status and age identification. *American Sociological Review, 21,* 201.

Blau, Z. S. (1973). Aging, widowhood, and retirement: A sociological perspective. In Z. Blau (Ed.), *Old age in a changing society* (pp. 21–36). New York: Franklin Watts.

Bock, E. W. (1972). Aging and suicide. *Family Coordinator, 21,* 71–79.

Bock, E. W., & Webber, I. L. (1972). Suicide among the elderly: Isolating and mitigating alternatives. *Journal of Marriage and the Family, 34,* 24–31.

Booth, A. (1972). Sex and social participation. *American Sociological Review, 37,* 183–193.

Bornstein, P. E., Clayton, P. J., Halikas, J. A., Maurice, W. L., & Rogins, E. (1973). The depression of widowhood after 13 months. *British Journal of Psychiatry, 122,* 561.

Botwinick, J. (1973). *Aging and behavior.* New York: Springer.

Breed, W. (1963). Occupational mobility and suicide among white males. *American Sociological Review, 28,* 179–188.

Breed, W., & Huffine, C. L. (1979). Sex differences among older white Americans: A role and developmental approach. In O. Kaplan (Ed.), *Psychopathology of aging* (pp. 289–309). New York: Academic Press.

Bromley, D. B. (1966). *The psychology of human aging.* Baltimore: Penquin.

Burvil, P. W. (1972). Recent decreased ratio of male-female suicide rates. *International Journal of Social Psychiatry, 18,* 137–139.

Busse, E. W., & Pfeiffer, E. (1969). Functional psychiatric disorders in old age. In E. W. Busse & E. Pfeiffer (Eds.), *Behavior and adaptation in late life* (pp. 158–211). Boston: Little, Brown & Co.

Butler, R. N. (1975). *Why survive? Being old in America.* New York: Harper & Row.

Caine, L. (1974). *Widow.* New York: William Morrow & Co.

Cavan, R. S. (1928). *Suicide.* New York: Russell & Russell.

Clayton, P. J., Halikas, J. A., & Maurice, W. L. (1971). The bereavement of the widowed. *Diseases of the Nervous System, 32,* 597–604.

Cohen, F., & Lazarus, R. (1979). Coping with the stresses of illness. In G. Stone, F. Cohen, & N. Adler (Eds.), *Health and psychology: A handbook* (pp. 217–255). San Francisco: Jossey-Bass.

Cowgill, D. O., & Holmes, L. D. (Eds.). (1972). *Aging and modernization.* New York: Appleton-Century-Crofts.

Dohrenwend, B. S., & Dohrenwend, B. P. (Eds.). (1974). *Stressful life events: Their nature and effects.* New York: John Wiley & Sons.

Dorpat, T. L., Anderson, W. F., & Ripley, H. S. (1968). The relationship of physical illness to suicide. In H. L. P. Resnik (Ed.), *Suicidal behaviors: Diagnosis and management* (pp. 209–219). Boston: Little, Brown & Co.

Dotson, F. (1951). Patterns of voluntary association among urban working class families. *American Sociological Review, 16,* 687–693.

Dovenmuehle, R. H., & Verwoerdt, A. (1962). Physical illness and depressive symptomatology II. Factors of length of stay and severity of illness and frequency of hospitalization. *Journal of Gerontology, 18,* 260–266.

Dublin, L. I. (1963). *Suicide.* New York: Ronald Press.

Dublin, L. J., & Bunzel, B. (1933). *To be or not to be.* New York: Harrison, Smith & Robert Haas.

Dubovsky, S. L. (1978). Averting suicide in terminally ill patients. *Psychosomatics, 19,* 113–115.

Durkheim, E. (1951). *Suicide.* New York: Free Press. (Original work published 1897)

Durkheim, E. (1964). *The division of labor in society* (G. Simpson, Trans.). New York: Free Press. (Original work published 1933)

Eisdorfer, C., & Wilkie, F. (1977). Stress, disease, aging and behavior. In J. E. Birren & K. W. Schaie (Eds.), *Handbook of the psychology of aging* (pp. 251–275). New York: Van Nostrand Reinhold.

Falret, J. P. (1822). *De l'hypochondrie et du suicide.* Paris: Crouillebois.

Farber, M. L. (1968). *Theory of suicide.* New York: Funk & Wagnalls.

Farberow, N. L., & Moriwaki, S. (1975). Self-destructive crises in the older person. *Gerontologist, 15,* 333–337.

Freud, S. (1955). Mourning and melancholia. In J. Strachey (Ed.), *The standard edition of the complete works of Sigmund Freud* (pp. 247–252). London: Hogarth Press. (Original work published 1917)

Freud, S. (1955). Beyond the pleasure principle. In J. Strachey (Ed.) *The standard edition of the complete works of Sigmund Freud* (Vol. 18). London: Hogarth Press. (Original work published 1920).

Gardner, E. A., Bahn, A. K., & Mack, J. (1964). Suicide and psychiatric care in the aging. *Archives of General Psychiatry, 10,* 547–553.

Gibbs, J. P. (Ed.). (1965). *Suicide.* New York: Russell & Russell.

Giddens, A. (Ed.). (1971). *The sociology of suicide.* London: Frank Cass & Co.

Glick, I., Weiss, R., & Parkes, C. M. (1974). *The first year of bereavement.* New York: John Wiley & Sons.

Gubrium, J. F. (1974). Marital desolation and the evaluation of everyday life in old age. *Journal of Marriage and the Family,* 107–113.

Halbwachs, M. (1930) *Les causes du suicide.* Paris: Alcan.

Henry, A., & Short, J. F. (1954). *Suicide and homicide.* Glencoe, Ill.: Free Press.

Holmes, J., & Masuda, M. (1974). Life change and illness susceptibility. In B. Dohrenwend & B. Dohrenwend (Eds.), *Stressful life events* (pp. 45–73). New York: John Wiley & Sons.

Holmes, T. H., & Rahe, R. H. (1967). The social readjustment scale. *Journal of Psychosomatic Research, 11,* 213–218.

Hughes, E. C. (1981). *Men and their work.* Westport, Conn.: Greenwood.

Jarvik, L. E. (1975). Thoughts on the psychobiology of aging. *American Psychologist, 30,* 576–583.

Johnson, B. (1965). Durkheim's one cause of suicide. *American Sociological Review, 30*(6), 875–876.

Kaplan, O. J. (Ed.). (1979). *Psychopathology of aging.* New York: Academic Press.

Kastenbaum, R. (1964). The crisis of explanation. In R. Kastenbaum (Ed.), *New thoughts on old age* (pp. 316–323). New York: Springer.

Kastenbaum, R., & Aisenberg, R. (1972). *The psychology of death.* New York: Springer.

Kay, D. W., & Walk, A. (Eds.). (1971). Recent developments in psycho-geriatrics. *British Journal of Psychiatry* (Special publication) *6,* 1–113.

Kierkegaard, S. (1941). *The sickness unto death.* Princeton, N.J.: Princeton University Press. (Original work published 1849)

Kimmel, D. (1974). *Adulthood and aging.* New York: John Wiley & Sons.

Kobler, A. L., & Stotland, E. (1964). *The end of hope.* New York: Free Press.

Kopell, B. S. (1977). Treating the suicidal patient. *Geriatrics, 32,* 65–67.

Kramer, M., Pollack, E., Redick, R., & Locke, B. (1972). *Mental disorders: Suicide.* Cambridge, Mass.: Harvard University Press.

Kreitman, N. (1977). *Parasuicide.* New York: John Wiley & Sons.

Lauter, H. (1973). Altersdepressionen-ursachen Epidemiologie Nosologie. *Actuelle Gerontologie, 3,* 247–252.

Lazarus, R. S. (1966). *Psychological stress and the coping process.* New York: McGraw-Hill.

Lecky, W. E. H. (1869). *History of European morals from Augustus to Charlemagne* (2 vols.). New York: D. Appleton & Co.

Lehr, U. (1981). Stereotypes of aging and age norms. In D. Danon, N.W. Shock, and N. Maroes (Eds.), *Proceedings of the World Conference of Institute de la Vie. Vol 3, Aging: A challenge to science and society* (pp. 101–112). Oxford, England: Oxford University Press.

Lindemann, E. (1944). Symptomatology and management of acute grief. *American Journal of Psychiatry, 101*(2), 141–148.

Loether, H. J. (1975). *Problems of aging: Sociological and social psychological perspectives* (2nd ed.). Belmont, Calif.: Dickerson Publishing Co.

Lonnqvist, J. (1977). *Suicide in Helsinki* (Monographs on Psychiatry). Helsinki: Fennica.

Lopata, H Z. (1973). Self-identity in marriage and widowhood. *Sociological Quarterly, 14,* 407–418.

Lowenthal, M., & Haven, C. (1968). Interaction and adaptation: Intimacy as a critical variable. In B. Neugarten (Ed.), *Middle age and aging* (pp. 390–400). Chicago: University of Chicago Press.

Lynn, R. (1969). National rates of economic growth, anxiety, and suicide. *Nature, 222,* 494.

MacMahon, B., & Pugh, T. (1965). Suicide in the widowed. *American Journal of Epidemiology, 81,* 23–31.

Maris, R. W. (1967). Suicide, status, and mobility in Chicago. *Social Forces, 46,* 246–256.

Maris, R. W. (1969a). *Social forces in urban suicide.* Homewood, IL: Dorsey Press.

Maris, R. W. (1969b). The sociology of suicide prevention: Policy implications of differences between suicidal patients and completed suicides. *Social Problems, 17,* 133–149.

Marshall, J. R. (1978). Changes in aged white male suicide: 1948–1972. *Journal of Gerontology, 33,* 763–768.

McIntosh, J. L., Hubbard, R. W., & Santos, J. F. (1981). Suicide among the elderly: A review of issues with case studies. *Journal of Gerontological Social Work, 4*(1), 63–74.

McIntosh, J. L., & Santos, J. F. (1981). Suicide among minority elderly: A preliminary investigation. *Suicide and Life Threatening Behavior, 11,* 151–166.

Melville, H. (1964). *Moby Dick.* New York: Airmont.

Menninger, K. (1938). *Man against himself.* New York: Harcourt, Brace & World.

Miller, M. (1976). *Suicide among older men.* Unpublished doctoral dissertation, University of Michigan, Ann Arbor.

Miller, M. (1978). Toward a profile of the older white male suicide. *Gerontologist, 18,* 80–82.

Miller, M. (1979). *Suicide after sixty: The final alternative.* New York: Springer.

Miller, S. J. (1965). The social dilemma of the aging leisure participant. In A. M. Rose & W. A. Peterson (Eds.), *Older people and their social world* (77–92). Philadelphia: F. A. Davis.

Mizruchi, E. H. (1964). *Success and opportunity.* Glencoe, Ill.: Free Press.

Mizruchi, E. H. (1982). Abeyance process and time: An exploratory approach to age and social structure. In E. Mizruchi, B. Glassner, & T. Pastorello (Eds.), *Time and aging* (pp. 112–128). Bayside, N.Y.: General Hall.

Morselli, E. (1979). *Suicide.* New York: Appleton. (Original work published in 1882)

Murphy, G. E., & Robins, E. (1967). Social factors in suicide. *Journal of the American Medical Association, 199,* 303–308.

Neugarten, B. (Ed.). (1968). *Middle age and aging.* Chicago: University of Chicago Press.

Niccolini, R. (1973). Reading the signals for suicidal risk. *Geriatrics, 28,* 71–72.

O'Neal, P., Robins, E., & Schmidt, E. H. (1956). A psychiatric study of attempted suicide in persons over sixty years of age. *Archives of Neurological Psychiatry, 75,* 275–284.

Palmore, E., & Manton, K. (1974). Modernization and status of the aged: International correlations. *Journal of Gerontology, 29,* 205–210.

Parkes, C. M. (1965). Bereavement and mental illness. *British Journal of Medical Psychiatry, 38,* 1–26.

Paykel, E. S., Prusoff, B. A., & Myers, J. K. (1975). Suicide attempts and recent life events. *Archives of General Psychiatry, 32,* 327–333.

Payne, E. C. (1975). Depression and suicide. In J. G. Howells (Ed.), *Modern perspectives in the psychiatry of old age* (pp. 290–312). New York: Brunner/Mazel.

Pfeiffer, E. (1977). Psychopathology and social pathology. In J. E. Birren & K. W. Schaie (Eds.), *Handbook of the psychology of aging* (pp. 650–671). New York: Van Nostrand Reinhold.

Phillips, B. S. (1957). A role theory approach to adjustment in old age. *American Sociological Review, 22,* 212–217.

Powell, E. H. (1958). Occupation, status, and suicide. *American Sociological Review, 23*(2), 131–139.

Powell, E. H. (1970). *The design of discord.* New York: Oxford University Press.

Quinney, R. (1965). Suicide, homicide and economic development. *Social Forces, 43,* 401–408.

Rabkin, S. G., & Streuning, E. L. (1976). Life events, stress and illness. *Science, 194,* 1013–1020.

Rachlis, D. (1970). Suicide and loss adjustment in the aging. *Bulletin of Suicidology, 10,* 23–26.

Resnik, H. L. P., & Cantor, J. M. (1970). Suicide and aging. *Journal of the American Geriatric Society, 18,* 152–158.

Rosow, I. (1967). *Social integration of the aged.* New York: Free Press.

Rosow, I. (1973). The social context of the aging self. *Gerontologist, 12,* 82–87.

Sainsbury, P. (1955). *Suicide in London: An ecological study.* London: Chapman & Hall.

Sainsbury, P. (1962). Suicide in later life. *Gerontologica Clinica, 4,* 161–170.

Sainsbury, P. (1963). Social and epidemiological aspects of suicide with special reference to the aged. In R. H. Williams, C. Tibbitts, & W. Donahue (Eds.), *Processes of aging: Social and psychological perspectives* (Vol. 2, pp. 151–176). New York: Atherton.

Sainsbury, P., Walk, D., & Grad, J. (1966). Evaluating the Graylingwall hospital community psychiatric services in Chichester: Suicide and community care. *Milbank Memorial Fund Quarterly, 44*(1), 231–290.

Sainsbury, P. (1968). Suicide and depression. *British Journal of Psychiatry* (Special publication), *2,* 1–13.

Sainsbury, P. (1973). Suicide: Opinions and Parts. *Proceedings of the Royal Society of Medicine,* *66,* 579–587.

Salzman, C., & Shader, R. (1979). Clinical evaluation of depression in the elderly. In A. Raskin & L. Jarvik (Eds.), *Psychiatric symptoms and cognitive loss in the elderly* (pp. 39–57). New York: Hemisphere.

Schmid, C. F. (1928). *Suicide in Seattle 1914–1925: An ecological and behavioristic study.* Seattle: University of Washington Press.

Schulz, R. (1976). Effects of control and predictability on the physical and psychological well-being of the institutionalized aged. *Journal of Personality and Social Psychology, 33,* 563–573.

Seiden, R. (1981). Mellowing with age: Factors influencing the nonwhite suicide rate. *International Journal of Aging and Human Development, 13*(4), 265–281.

Seiden, R. (1983, November). *Suicide among the young and the elderly.* Paper presented at the annual meeting of the Gerontological Society of America, San Francisco, Calif.

Seligman, M. E. P. (1975). *Helplessness.* San Francisco: W. H. Freeman.

Seligman, M. E. P. (1976). Learned helplessness and depression in animals and men. In J. T. Spence, R. C. Carsen, & J. W. Thibaut (Eds.), *Behavioral approaches to therapy* (pp. 111–126). Morristown, N.J.: General Learning Press.

Selye, H. (1946). The general adaptation syndrome and the diseases of adaptation. *Journal of Clinical Endocrinology, 6,* 117–230.

Selye, H. (1955). General physiology and pathology of stress. In H. Selye & G. Heuser (Eds.), *5th Annual Report on Stress, 1955–56* (pp. 25–103). New York: Medical Publications.

Selye, H. (1956). *The stress of life.* New York: McGraw-Hill.

Selye, H. (1974). *Stress without distress.* Philadelphia: J. P. Lippincott.

Selye, H. (1976). *Stress in health and disease.* Boston: Butterworth.

Sendbuehler, J. M., & Goldstein, S. (1977). Attempted suicide among the aged. *Journal of the American Geriatric Society, 25,* 245–248.

Shanas, E., Townsend, P., Wedderburn, D., Friis, H., Milkof, P., Stehower, G. (Eds.), *Old people in three industrial societies.* New York: Atherton Press.

Shapiro, L. B. (1935). Suicide: Psychology and family tendency. *Journal of Nervous and Mental Diseases, 81,* 547.

Shneidman, E. S., & Farberow, N. L. (1957). *Clues to suicide.* New York: McGraw-Hill.

Stekel, W. (1918). On suicide. *American Journal of Urology and Sexology, 14,* 337–350.

Stengel, E. (1964). *Suicide and attempted suicide.* London: Penquin.

Stengel, E., & Cook, G. (1961). Contrasting suicide rates in industrial communities. *Journal of Mental Science, 107,* 1011.

Stone, G., Cohen, F., & Adler, N. (Eds.). (1979). *Health and psychology: A handbook.* San Francisco: Jossey-Bass.

Thompson, G. (1973). Work vs. leisure roles: An investigation of morale among employed and retired men. *Journal of Gerontology, 28,* 339–344.

Townsend, P. (1968). Isolation, desolation, and loneliness. In E. Shanas, P. Townsend, D. Wedderbury, H. Frus, P. Milkof, & G. Stehower (Eds.), *Old people in three industrial societies* (pp. 258–287). New York: Atherton Press.

Troll, L. E., Israel, J., & Israel, K. (1977). *Looking ahead: A woman's guide to the problems and joys of growing older.* Englewood Cliffs, N.J.: Prentice Hall.

Tunstall, J. (1966). *Old and alone: A sociological study of old people.* London: Routledge & Keagan Paul.

U. S. Bureau of the Census. (1980). *Statistical Abstract of the U. S.* (101 ed.). Washington, D.C.: U. S. Government Printing Office.

U. S. Bureau of the Census. (1982). *Statistical Abstract of the U. S., 1982–83* (103 ed.). Washington, D.C.: U. S. Government Printing Office.

Vachon, M. S. (1976). Grief and bereavement following the death of a spouse. *Canadian Psychiatric Association Journal, 21,* 35–43.

Weigert, A. J., & Hastings, R. (1977). Identity loss, family, and social change. *American Journal of Sociology, 82*(6), 1171–1185.

Weiss, J. M. A. (1968). Suicide in the aged. In H. L. P. Resnik (Ed.), *Suicidal behaviors: Diagnosis and management* (pp. 255–267). Boston: Little, Brown & Co.

Welford, A. T. (1962). On changes of performance with age. *Lancet, 1,* 335–339.

Williams, R. M., Jr. (1970). *American society.* New York: Knopf.

Winokur, G. (1974, November). Lecture given at the Clark Institute of Psychiatry, Toronto, Canada.

Wolff, K. (1971). The treatment of the depressed and suicidal geriatric patient. *Geriatrics, 26,* 65–69.

Part I

Suicide Susceptibility:
Diagnosis and Assessment

Chapter 1

A Profile of the "At-Risk" Elderly

INTRODUCTION

The joint suicide of Karl Marx's daughter and her husband, Dr. Paul Lafargue, took place in 1911. The gardener discovered their bodies in a room off the garden of their home in Paris. "He was lying fully dressed on a bed; she was in an easy chair in an adjoining room. Before committing suicide Dr. Lafargue had written out a reference for his domestic help, signed his will, and even drafted the text of a telegram to be sent to his nephew (announcing their deaths)" (Choron, 1972, p. 100). In his suicide note to friends, Lafargue said:

> Sound of mind and body, I am killing myself before pitiless old age, which gradually deprives me of the pleasures and joys of existence and saps my physical and intellectual forces, will paralyze my energy, break my will power, and turn me into a burden to myself and others. Long ago I have promised myself not to live beyond the age of seventy. I have fixed the moment for my departure from life and I have prepared the method of executing my project: a hypodermic injection of hydrocyanic acid. (Choron, 1972, p. 100)

In 1975, Dr. and Mrs. Henry P. Van Dusen, aged 77 and 80 respectively, attempted suicide by taking an overdose of sleeping pills. Mrs. Van Dusen died immediately. Dr. Van Dusen survived but died two weeks later of a heart ailment. The Van Dusens were well-known figures in American religion. Before his retirement, Dr. Van Dusen had been president of Union Theological Seminary and a prominent ecumenical leader. The couple's decision to commit suicide was evidently the result of long and thoughtful reflection. Both Van Dusens were members of the Euthanasia Society and, according to the *New York Times* report, "had entered into the [suicide] pact rather than face the prospect of debilitating old age." In the suicide note left by them, they explicitly vowed that they would not "die in a nursing home." Both Van Dusens suffered from chronic health problems: she from arthritis, he from the effects of a stroke that interfered with normal speech. The *Times* report noted that, "for the vigorous articulate Presbyterian scholar and his active wife, the setbacks were serious impediments to living the kind of useful, productive lives to which they had become accustomed" (Briggs, 1975, p. 1). Both suicides reflected a rational decision to end life rather than face a decreased quality of life and the pain and suffering of old age.

When Socrates drank the hemlock at age 70, he offered as one reason for his death the fact that he was old. Later, Stoic philosophers reaffirmed that the ultimate criterion of a "good life" should be quality, not quantity, thus rationalizing suicide on the grounds of old age.

DOCUMENTED CASES OF ELDERLY SUICIDE

In this section we present actual cases of completed or potential geriatric suicide drawn from our own research experience and from studies and analyses of other professional observers. The first five cases are from our own research, based on analyses of suicide notes and discussions with spouses, relatives, and friends of elderly suicide victims.

1. Mr. A's wife had terminal cancer. She had been in and out of hospitals several times during the year in which she died. Mr. A was very close to his wife and spent all his time nursing her when she was at home. When she died, he was grief-stricken. He called the local office on aging and cried on the phone for an hour. The next morning a social worker found Mr. A dead in his home. The coroner's report cited a mixture of drugs and alcohol as the cause of death.

2. Mr. B had lived with his wife in a mobile home retirement community on Florida's "Gold Coast." In our conversation, Mrs. B painfully related the story of her husband's recent suicide. According to his widow, Mr. B had always been a jovial, happy-go-lucky man with an unsurpassed enthusiasm for life. He loved working in the yard, making home repairs, and fishing. About six months before his suicide, Mr. B had undergone coronary bypass surgery, during which he stopped breathing, his heart stopped beating, and he was pulseless. Although his vital functions

returned and the surgeons completed the operation successfully, Mr. B was a changed man afterward. He became sullen and bitter, refused to go out or do anything, got angry at the smallest incidents, and flew into rages during which he yelled, screamed, and threw things. Mrs. B was frightened of him. She described him as totally irrational and unpredictable, adding, "Something happened on that operating table; my husband was totally transformed, and I didn't know him." One evening, six months after the operation, Mr. B disappeared. The next morning his body was found several miles from home. He had shot himself in the head.

3. Mrs. C lived alone in a condominium in a retirement community. Late one night she threw herself into a lagoon and drowned. Neighbors reported that shortly before her death Mrs. C had become sad and depressed, refusing to talk to anyone and always looking "down in the mouth." In the few days immediately preceding her death, she had remained in her home, seeing no one.

4. Mr. D was a 72-year old physician. He was almost totally blind as a result of the progression of diabetes. He took an overdose of sleeping pills, leaving a suicide note in which he wrote, "If I cannot see, I cannot practice medicine. Medicine is my life. Without it I am dead, so I choose to end my life now."

5. Mr. E was a retired school teacher who killed himself shortly before his 69th birthday. In his suicide note to his ailing wife he wrote, "I can no longer provide for the two of us on my meager Social Security. At least through my death you can live on the insurance money. Please destroy this note, so you will collect the full insurance benefits. I love you."

The next two cases of potentially suicidal elderly (elderly who either attempted suicide or made statements of suicidal intent) come from the files of cases referred to the Help Outreach Program for the Elderly (HOPE), a peer counseling and outreach program to identify and help the frail and vulnerable elderly (McIntosh, Hubbard, & Santos, 1981).

1. *Mr. R, age 76: Rational Suicide*

Upon receiving a diagnosis of cancer with a recommendation for surgery that had a 50% success rate, Mr. R signed himself out of the hospital stating, "I do not want surgery. When the pain gets real bad, I'll take care of things myself." The doctor notified

HOPE, and a home visit was arranged the same day. Mr. R reported that his wife had died two years earlier of the same type of cancer and that surgery had served only to prolong her pain; it did not improve her health. He further stated, "I'm not crazy. My wife is gone, my kids are raised, I've lived a good life. I'm ready to die, I just don't want to go through much pain."

2. Mrs. W, age 67: Chronic Suicidal Behavior

Mrs. W had a history of chronic depression which had led to suicide attempts in middle age. At the age of 64 she made two more unsuccessful attempts, one shortly after the death of her husband and another four months later. After this last attempt she was institutionalized and referred to HOPE. Mrs. W's history included chronic depression and alcoholism, which seemed to interact in precipitating her suicidal attempts. Her later years of life had resulted in increased trauma and loss, which brought about increased suicidal behavior. HOPE workers participated in discharge planning for Mrs. W and continued weekly visits to her in her home. Six weeks after her discharge, Mrs. W's son was given a job transfer, moving him far away from his mother. When alerted to this new trauma, HOPE workers contacted Mrs. W's psychiatrist and began visiting her three times a week. A suicidal threat made by Mrs. W resulted in short-term institutionalization procedures.

While one does not generally think of suicidal behavior in terms of chronicity, it is clear that in many cases individuals who are predisposed to suicidal behavior may suffer losses and trauma in older age which increase the likelihood of suicidal attempts. In the second case described above, Mrs. W had three significant variations indicating a high suicidal risk: (1) prior attempts, (2) chronic depression and alcohol use, and (3) recent trauma and loss.

The final three cases are of completed suicides of elderly males reported by Miller (1979).*

1. Mr. A was the second of five children. He was described by his widow as a quiet person who continually had "a chip on his

shoulder." Someone was always "rubbing him the wrong way," especially his bosses, whom he "just about hated."

For many years Mr. A had acted "as though the world had done him wrong." When he was in business he would often "kick customers out and tell them to go to hell." He particularly disliked students or anyone with an education, which was unfortunate because he had lived for many years in a college town. When he was drunk, he would become violent and unpredictable.

The son of a domineering father, Mr. A was one-quarter American Indian. He had few friends but had been close to one of his brothers; however, his brother's death preceded his own by several years. When his mother died about three years before his suicide, he refused to attend her funeral because he claimed he was sicker than she had been.

Mr. A's father-in-law had tried to kill himself in 1924 and 1932. Both attempts were apparently the result of poor business conditions and in both cases he had slashed his wrists. It is not known what influence, if any, these acts ultimately had on his son-in-law. However, Mr. A also attempted suicide twice during a five-day period in 1969. The first attempt was with gas; the second involved drugs (although a gun was found near the body that had not been fired). No psychiatric services were obtained for Mr. A as a result of those incidents. He apparently gave no explanation for his actions, but his widow concluded, "He just got tired of taking pills." She said, "He had made it clear to me he didn't want a lingering death."

In 1950, Mr. A experienced the first of six heart attacks. The worst and final one took place in 1973, only a few months before his suicide. The doctors told his wife he had been dead for half an hour, but they were able to resuscitate him. Mrs. A was angry and asked the doctors, "Why didn't you just let him go?"

While being operated on for his heart condition, Mr. A suffered a stroke that left his right hand and the right side of his face paralyzed. The doctors told Mrs. A the stroke had been caused by "being on the heart-lung machine for too long." The operation was not completely successful and another was performed the following night to close a small artery that was still bleeding.

Mr. A also developed speech problems. His words would run together and sound like gibberish, and he would cry. After a complete physical examination, it was determined the problem was caused by his medication. His speech problem abated when the medicine was changed.

During the next few months Mr. A seemed unhappy and depressed, although he was responding well to physical therapy. Two weeks before his suicide, his physician examined him and reported he was "doing just great." A few days before his death at age 62, a physical therapist was unusually rough with him and he cried from the pain. Mrs. A felt that event was the catalyst for her husband's suicide, even though she believed he would have done it anyway sooner or later.

The night before his death, Mr. and Mrs. A had gone out to supper with another couple. They enjoyed themselves, and he seemed to his wife to be "at peace with the world and himself . . . somehow relieved." The couple even discussed spending the hot summer months up in the mountains, and Mr. A had agreed to join them. Giving no indication of what he was about to do, he awoke early the next morning and shot himself in the head.

2. After he became an alcoholic, Mr. I's first wife divorced him. Later he remarried and stopped drinking for 15 years. For no apparent reason—even Mr. I said he did not understand why—he suddenly began drinking again. His second wife, six years his senior, said that when he was not drinking he was an amiable and hard-working man.

For many years Mr. I had been a spray painter in a factory. The color of the paint he used last could be seen when he coughed into a handkerchief. Eventually he developed tuberculosis and was in a sanitarium for a year and a half, although several times he became angry and left without medical approval. The top lobe of his right lung was removed, and for the rest of his life he experienced difficulty breathing. For many years he had stomach problems, which had been diagnosed as ulcers; however; he suspected he had cancer of the stomach.

His employment history was checkered. Whenever he got angry on the job, he would quit.

Information about two previous suicide attempts was sketchy, but it appeared he swallowed arsenic about 30 years before his death and was saved by stomach pumping. About three years before his death, he swallowed 15 valiums and again had his stomach pumped. Throughout his adult life he often threatened suicide. Mr. I's mother died in a mental hospital. She had been institutionalized six times. Two of her brothers had also been in mental institutions, and another of Mr. I's uncles had killed himself.

Because of his chronic alcoholism, Mr. I was seeing a psychiatrist at the time of his suicide. Mr. I had previously been institutionalized for a week after he tried to shoot his wife. When he was drunk he would often beat her. Once he threatened her by saying, "I could go in there any night and choke you to death and there wouldn't be a thing you could do to stop me." On another occasion, he told her, "If I can't live with you, no one will." She finally grew tired of his abuse, separated from him and was suing for divorce at the time of his death.

When drunk Mr. I was not responsible for his actions. Twice he sold his automobiles to obtain money to buy alcohol; he sold one for $25. Besides smoking more than two packs of cigarettes a day for many years, he had become reliant on valium. Because of his chronic alcohol problem, he was receiving Social Security disability benefits.

A month before his death, Mr. I wrote a "To Whom It May Concern" letter and placed it in a tin box where he kept important papers. The letter contained instructions stating he did not want any funeral service, flowers, or obituary. He also said he wanted to be buried in a sport shirt and slacks, not a suit.

On the morning of his suicide, Mr. I came to his wife's home. He had obviously been drinking and had brought a half-filled bottle of liquor with him. He asked to see their dog and after petting it, went out on the steps in front of the house and laid down. He pulled out a gun and showed it to his wife. She struggled to get it away from him, but he still managed to shoot himself in the head. Because her hand was on the pistol when it fired, she received powder burns.

The last thing the 60-year-old Mr. I did before shooting himself was take a drink.

3. The product of a cruel father and a very unhappy childhood in Austria, Mr. N was already an alcoholic when he was 29 years old. After he beat his wife and she divorced him, he joined Alcoholics Anonymous. He had been sober for five years when he remarried the same woman. She described their life together as "so miserable it was like being in a concentration camp." They rarely, if ever, had intimate relations during either of their marriages.

Mr. N was a precise person who lived his entire life "by the minute and the second." Because he was obsessed with money, he refused to pay any of his wife's bills. She said "she took that for granted when she married him." He once told his wife that when he walked through the supermarket and saw how high the prices were he would "shiver and tremble all over."

Mr. N had been raised in a "suicidal family." While still living in Austria (a country with one of the highest suicide rates in the world), his grandfather, an uncle, an aunt, and his father had killed themselves. Mr. N's mother had seriously attempted suicide by trying to jump to her death. Mr. N spoke of his own suicide for many years. He told his stepdaughter, "my entire family killed themselves, so I must kill myself too." He told his wife he was afraid to have any children because of all the suicides in his family.

He had no friends, rarely smiled or laughed, and often wondered why he was born. He scoffed at humor on television, saying, "life is not humorous, and anyone who laughs about it is an idiot."

Mr. N never went to doctors because he didn't want to pay their fees. Five years before his suicide, he saw a therapist at a mental clinic, who said that Mr. N was obsessed with money. Mr. N never returned because he said the $3 fee charged for the hour sessions was too expensive.

Four years before his death, Mr. N lost $45,000 by investing in an apartment house. He was a serious gambler who studied horse racing "as though he were doing deep research." During the stock market decline in 1974, he lost $20,000 in various investments.

Shortly after his sister became widowed, Mrs. N suggested they invite the woman to move into their home. He agreed, but they both regretted their decision because he argued with his sister much of the time she lived with them.

Mr. N [previously] was a very healthy man, but he was diagnosed as having cancer of the pancreas and pronounced terminal. He was deeply troubled by the possibility his wife would die and leave him with the sister he hated.

In his last year, at the age of 67, Mr. N had begun to work part-time in a liquor store. He argued with many of the customers and was afraid of losing his job. He worried that he would not be able to find another job at his age, even though there was no financial need for him to work. Yet he was terrified of going to work because the same man had robbed the store three times. Because the robber threatened Mr. N with a gun, the manager purchased a pistol to be kept in the store for protection. That was the gun Mr. N used to kill himself.

A few days before he killed himself, he asked his stepdaughter if she had any sleeping pills. He told her he needed them because "I want to get out."

Nothing unusual happened the day of his suicide except he left his lunch at home. At lunchtime he shot himself in the head. His widow felt he was too methodical a man to have forgotten his lunch.

These real-life cases of completed or attempted suicide demonstrate the interplay of various suicidogenic forces in late life. Based on his studies of completed suicides of elderly males, Miller (1979) concluded that late-life suicide may be classified into one of eight patterns: (1) reaction to physical illness, (2) reaction to mental illness, (3) reaction to retirement, (4) reaction to death of a spouse, (5) reaction to threat of dependency or institutionalization, (6) pathological personal relationships, (7) alcoholism and drug abuse, or (8) multiple causes.

The cases we have presented highlight, in particular, the negative effects of loss of spouse, retirement, and physical illness and also the role of alcoholism and of early life experiences. Depression and mental health problems are common in geriatric suicides. Most of the cases reveal that suicide among the elderly most often represents a permanent solution to what is perceived to be, and may actually be, an intolerable life situation. The elderly kill themselves when life no longer has any meaning for them, when they feel helpless to alter present life conditions or the future, and when they retain no hope that things will improve. Unlike many younger individuals who choose suicide as a permanent solution to what in reality may be a temporary problem, the elderly usually choose suicide because the problems they face are not easily solvable.

Table 1–1, derived from a review of existing literature and from information obtained from actual case records of geriatric suicides, presents a profile of the "at-risk" elderly.

Table 1–1 Risk Factors in Elderly Suicide

Factor	High Risk	Low Risk
Sex	Male	Female
Religion	Protestant	Catholic or Jewish
Race	White	Nonwhite
Marital status	Widowed or divorced	Married
Occupational background	Blue collar, low-paying job Disorderly career Occupational skidding	Professional or white collar job Orderly career
Current employment status	Retired or unemployed	Employed full- or part-time

Living environment	Urban
	Living alone
	Isolated
	Recent move
		Rural
		Living with spouse or
		  other relatives
		Living in close-knit
		  neighborhood

Physical health	Poor health Terminal illness Pain and suffering	Good health

Mental health	Depression
	Alcoholism
	Low self-concept and
	  self-esteem
	Lonely
	Feeling rejected, unloved
		Happy and well-adjusted
		Positive self-concept
		Positive outlook on life
		Sense of competence and
		  personal control over life

Personal background	Broken home; rejecting,
	  critical parents; shy or
	  dependent personality;
	  history of poor inter-
	  personal relationships; a
	  "loner"; previous
	  depression.
	History of mental illness in
	  family, poor marital history,
	  poor work record, rigid,
	  tunnel vision, circular
	  reasoning
		Intact family-of-origin; warm,
		  loving parents; autonomous,
		  independent, and assertive;
		  flexible and adaptable;
		  history of close friendships,
		  no previous depression, no
		  history of mental illness in
		  family.
		No previous suicide
		  attempts, no history of
		  suicide in family, good
		  marital history, good work
		  record

REFERENCES

Briggs, K.A. (1975, February 26). Suicide pact precedes deaths of Dr. Van Dusen and his wife. *New York Times*, pp. 1, 43.

Choron, J. (1972). *Suicide*. New York: Charles Scribner & Sons.

McIntosh, J. L., Hubbard, R. W., & Santos, J. F. (1981). Suicide among the elderly: A review of issues with case studies. *Journal of Gerontological Social Work, 4*(1), 63–74.

Miller, M. (1979). *Suicide after sixty: The final alternative*. New York: Springer.

Chapter 2

Depression in the Elderly: Etiology and Assessment

Mary Lou Melville and Dan G. Blazer II

The term *depression* is an imprecise, confusing one, both for the public and for health care professionals. Yet it denotes a condition known and described for centuries. A current psychiatric definition of the most common central phenomenon in the feeling state of depression is "a dysphoric mood ... or loss of interest or pleasure in all or almost all usual activities or pastimes" (American Psychiatric Association, 1980). Dysphoria, from the Greek, meaning "excessive pain, anguish or agitation," is used in medical terminology to indicate "disquiet, restlessness, malaise" (Dorland's Illustrated Medical Dictionary, 25th ed.). This central dysphoric feeling is usually accompanied by a panoply of other feelings, signs, and symptoms that involve the entire spectrum of human woes—from a mild sense of disquiet to profound emptiness, melancholy, and despair. There have been efforts to understand the depressive condition. Are there many types of depression, or is the state indeed a single phenomenon, with many manifestations? Is depression a medical illness? A social or religious problem? Do some types of depression have roots in a malfunctioning soma while others arise solely from the *psyche*? Is depression a natural and unavoidable concomitant of old age? Numerous theories have evolved concerning these questions and continue to do so; however, there are as yet no definite answers.

In this chapter, our discussion focuses on some points and problems concerning depression, particularly depression in the elderly. Etiological theories of depressive illness are multitudinous; however, only a few of them are examined here. Finally, the evaluation and assessment of depression in late life are considered.

Mary Lou Melville, M.D., is Clinical Instructor of Psychiatry, Department of Psychiatry, Duke University Medical Center, Durham, North Carolina. Dan G. Blazer II, M.D., Ph.D., heads the Division of Social and Community Psychiatry, Duke University Medical Center, Durham, North Carolina.

14

PSYCHOSOCIAL THEORIES

During the past century, numerous psychosocial theories of depression, including depression in the aged, have been advanced. As divergent as these theories are, stemming from many different investigative areas, they have points of convergence. Many of the psychosocial theories of late-life depression center around the coexistence of two factors: stress, especially that of loss, combined with an individual's personal rigidity or lack of adaptability. In these theories, the tremendous stresses of the senium are seen as a forceful threat to the elder's emotional equilibrium. The person who does not have, or has lost, the ability to balance needs and losses is the one who will become depressed.

Freud and other early psychoanalysts asserted that maladjusted childhood patterns of development persist throughout human life and are the cause of abnormal behavior. Although analysts believe that many persons are capable of changing these patterns through psychoanalytic treatment, Freud (1924) himself believed that after the age of around 50, the "elasticity of the mental processes" had, as a rule, vanished and that older persons could no longer be taught to modify their behavior through treatment. With character structure fixed, Freud's elder must encounter the losses of old age. Freud also drew the connection between normal mourning and melancholia (severe depression), noting that although loss, either real or imagined, was a common factor in both conditions, that in melancholia there was an inability to acquiesce and accept loss in the normal way. He postulated that an imbalance of the usual ambivalent feelings toward any object led to turning the negative, aggressive impulses toward the self, creating guilt and depression (Freud, 1957). Erickson (1959) and Zetzel (1965) also indicate that the lack of certain qualities, including acceptance and a kind of flexible passivity, can lead to despair and depression in old age. Cath (1965) speaks of the "depletion anxiety" of old age, in which the balance of various psychic energies is enormously stressed by the losses of aging. The greater the imbalance of these forces, the greater the depression and despair. Levine (1965) notes that, not only external losses, but one's own feelings and perceptions can evoke a dramatic intrapsychic disequilibrium, leading to depression. In Klein's (1948) theory of the depressive position, in Bibring's (1953) work on self-esteem, in Beck's (1967) theory of negative self-concept, and in other works, the theme recurs that early experiences, and the subject's reactions to them, set patterns of response that are maladaptive in new situations and lead to feelings of low self-esteem, self-hatred, and emptiness. In many of these theories, such patterns are seen as becoming clinically evident only when tremendous stress, such as that of old age, causes a breakdown of marginally adequate coping. On the other hand, Blau and Berezin (1975) theorize that nonadaptive response patterns can, indeed, arise *de novo* in late life, triggered by a pattern of repetitive failures and losses. Spitz (1946) observed "anaclitic" (from the Greek for leaning) depression in infants separated from their mothers. He theorized that the overwhelming loss, to which the infants could not accommodate, led to depression. The most severe form of anaclitic depression is manifested by a syndrome now called "failure to thrive," which may culminate in death. Blau (1980) has pointed out that the decline and death of aged persons soon after entering a long-term care facility could be equated with anaclitic depression.

BIOLOGICAL AND GENETIC THEORIES

In the latter half of this century, there has been a resurgence of biological theories of depression. One such theory, the catecholamine hypothesis of affective disorders, is based, in part, on evidence that certain drugs either potentiate or increase catecholamine neurotransmitters involved in brain activity. These same drugs, notably the MAO-inhibiters and tricyclic antidepressants, also have an antidepressant effect. In addition, drugs that tend to diminish the activity of neurotransmitters, such as reserpine, also sedate or depress. The theory, summarized by Schildkraut (1965), states that at least some depressions are associated with a deficiency of catecholamines (especially norepinephrine) at important receptor sites in the brain. Another biogenic amine theory involves the neurotransmitter serotonin. Studies have demonstrated abnormally low levels and activity of a serotonin metabolite in the spinal fluid of some depressive patients. Van Praag (1982) has noted that such patients have a greater family history of depression than those without the abnormality. His study also demonstrated an unusually high incidence of completed suicide, at one year follow-up, in both depressed and previously suicidal patients with the abnormality. Other studies demonstrate a serotonin disorder both in persons who have committed violent offenses and in those who have attempted violent suicide (Brown, Goodwin, Ballenger, Goyer, & Major, 1979). These associations, found in biological research, are reminiscent of those that link depression, aggression, and anger in numerous psychosocial theories.

A correlate of the biogenic amine theory is the endocrine theory of depression. This theory attributes depressive illness to disorders in complex connections between the pituitary gland, the hypothalamic nuclei of the brain, and endocrine organs (such as the thyroid and adrenal glands). An example of the research evidence for this theory involves the secretion of the growth hormone (GH) by the pituitary. GH is secreted by humans of all ages; its level in the blood is elevated in response to several factors, including stress. Numerous GH stimulation studies have demonstrated that many depressed persons have a diminished GH response level. Inhibited GH response has also been found in maternal deprivation and in the "failure to thrive" syndrome, the same condition as the endstage of Spitz's (1946) anaclitic depression.

Other aspects of the endocrine theory involve both cortisol and thyroid-stimulating hormones (TSH). Many depressed patients have been found to hypersecrete cortisol; moreover, depressives frequently cannot "turn off" cortisol secretion normally. Other depressed subjects have abnormally low responses to attempted stimulation of TSH. These observations have led to new diagnostic tests for depression, which will be discussed later.

Genetic theories of depression are based, in part, on studies showing increased risk for affective disorders, primarily manic-depressive types, in genetically related persons. A possible genetic contribution to old age depression may involve mechanisms that contribute to the brain cell loss observed in some aged persons (Blazer, 1982). Such cell loss affects several brain areas, including the locus ceruleus, an area that Hartmann (1973) has noted to be especially important in regulating norepinephrine systems and controlling rapid eye movement (REM) sleep, the sleep phase most disordered in severe depression.

Many biological theories, as well as psychosocial ones, emphasize a systems imbalance in the depressed person, that is, a failure of psychophysiologic adaptive mechanisms during stress. Perhaps the two kinds of theories are similar because the well-described behaviors observed by psychosocial theorists may indeed be congruent with actual pathophysiological events. Freud and his fellow analysts of the nineteenth century believed in the concept of "mind-body isomorphism" (McCarley & Hobson, 1977), that is, mind and body follow the same basic rules, as manifested in macro- and microphenomena. Biopsychosocial researchers are gradually finding links between behaviors and neurochemical events; someday they may perhaps discover the underlying rules.

THE NATURE OF DEPRESSION

Who Is Depressed?—The Clinician's View

Clinicians have traditionally described depression by studying patients—persons who come, or are brought, for treatment. They have, for the most part, tended to differentiate between two major groups of depressive subjects on the basis of symptoms, signs, and clinical history. One group has been termed variously as clinical, primary, endogenous, major, vital, psychotic, or physiological. Criteria for this group have varied somewhat but in general, have included relatively greater severity; occur either with or without a prior stressful event; signs and symptoms of disordered bodily functions (such as severe sleeping and digestive disorder); and symptoms of hallucinations, delusions, and disordered thought. More recently, this group of subjects has generally been found to be the one more responsive to biological therapies, such as antidepressant drugs and electroconvulsive therapy (ECT). The second group of depressive subjects has been called secondary, exogenous, minor, or reactive. Depression in this group has been considered to be less severe, to occur in reaction to events, to have both less body function disorder and no psychotic symptoms, and to show less response to biologic therapy. Indeed, some suggest that depression is not the proper term to describe such symptoms, choosing terms such as demoralization or "decreased life satisfaction." The dividing line between the two groups has been unclear; both elderly and suicidal depressions may fall into either diagnostic category.

Confusion concerning depressive diagnosis has made scientific study of the condition difficult, leading to increased efforts to define and quantify diagnostic criteria, using clinical and laboratory data. The diagnostic criteria in widest clinical use today are those in the third edition of the *Diagnostic and Statistical Manual of Mental Disorders* (DSM III) (American Psychiatric Association, 1980). This manual divides depression into the following categories: bipolar disorder (formerly manic-depressive), major depression (both single-episode and recurrent), dysthymic disorder (formerly depressive neurosis), and cyclothymic disorder. In addition, there are numerous other disorders that must be considered in differential diagnosis of elderly depression. There continues to be debate among clinicians over depressive classifications; DSM III will be updated and revised in the future as clinical and research experience dictate. The manual is written with a minimum of technical terms and contains a great deal of detailed diagnostic information. Any reader interested in geriatric depression is strongly encouraged to become familiar with this work.

The Epidemiology of Late-Life Depression

Further confusing the problem of "Who is depressed?" are data from psychiatric epidemiologists. They have approached the problem by surveying the general population, not patients, for depressive symptoms. Not surprisingly, a different picture emerges from this work. Many studies have demonstrated, as did Boyd, Weissman, Thompson, and Myers (1982), that at any given time a majority of the U.S. population has one or two depressive symptoms. Indeed, between 9 and 20 percent of the population has enough symptoms to score in the "depressed" range on self-report depression symptom scales. However, if clinical diagnostic instruments are used in the same population, the prevalence of depressive disorder is estimated at only 3 percent for men and just over 4 percent for women, indicating that there is a large group of persons who are suffering significantly but do not fall into a category of clinically diagnosable depression. In geriatric population surveys, rates of significant depressive symptoms in the elderly, estimated by use of symptom checklists, range from 10 to 45 percent. However, studies using clinical psychiatric evaluations have indicated that the prevalence of major and minor depression in older populations is only between 2 and 5 percent (Blazer, 1982). These studies would seem to indicate that, although the prevalence of diagnosable *depression* is not much greater in the elderly than in the general population, the group of elderly persons who suffer significant depressive *symptoms* may indeed be larger. Seemingly congruent with this observation is the fact that persons over 60 years old have the highest rate of suicide of any group in the United States. Therefore, it is only with humility, and a plan of constant reassessment, that anyone can presume to answer the question, "who is depressed?"

EVALUATION OF DEPRESSION

Initial Interview

In discussing evaluation of an older person for depressive symptoms, it must be stressed that anyone with a social or professional role in the elder's life can make a good initial assessment. The best evaluations are by persons who feel genuine interest and concern and who repeatedly observe the elder over time and in depth.

The older person should first be interviewed alone, if possible. Next, the assessor should meet with family and other informants. Finally the elder and the elder's supporting network should be evaluated together. The assessor should be alert for factors that can impede the initial interview. Among these are anxieties, sensory impairments (especially hearing loss), suspicions, and preconceived ideas about the interview. As Blazer (1982) notes, the interviewer should be prepared to proceed at a clam's pace, speaking slowly and distinctly. Sitting close to, or touching, an anxious older person may be reassuring; many elders do not have the same inhibitions about touch as younger ones (Blazer, 1982). Some subjects, however, may feel that touching implies disrespect. An older person should be addressed by surname with the appropriate title (Mr., Miss, etc.) unless the person requests that the first name be used. As older persons often make omissions in an interview, active inquiries should be made about each area of concern. Close observation of the elder is important. Nonverbal communications may often reveal whether tension, fears, or misunderstandings are developing. In addition, many of the observable signs of depression (see Table 2–1) may be evident, even though the subject offers no depressive complaints.

Table 2-1 Symptoms and Signs of Late-Life Depression

Symptoms	*Signs*
Emotional: Sad, dejected, decreased life satisfaction; loss of interest, impulse to cry, irritable, fearful, anxious, worried. Sense of hopelessness, helplessness, failure, emptiness, loneliness, uselessness. Negative feelings toward self.	*Appearance*: Stooped, sad, hostile, crying, whining, anxious, irritable, suspicious, uncooperative, socially withdrawn.
Cognitive: Low self-esteem, self-criticism, pessimism, suicidal thoughts, ruminations, doubt of values, concentration and memory difficulty. Delusions: uselessness, blame, somatic, nihilistic. Hallucinations: auditory, visual, kinesthetic.	*Examination*: Weight loss, confusion, clouding of consciousness, mood variation, bowel impaction. *Severe cases*: Drooling, unkempt appearance, ulcerations of skin or cornea due to picking, decreased blinking.
Physical: Loss of appetite and libido, fatigable, initial and terminal insomnia, frequent awakenings, constipation, pain, restlessness.	*Psychomotor retardation*: Slowed speech, movements, gait; minimal gestures. *Severe cases*: Muteness, stupor, semicoma; cessation of chewing, swallowing, blinking.
Volitional: Loss of motivation, inability to get going, "paralysis of will."	*Psychomotor agitation*: pacing, restlessness, hand wringing, picking at skin, constant motor activity, grasping at others.
	Unusual behavior: suicidal gestures, negativism, refusal to eat or drink, aggressive outbursts, stiffness, falling backwards.

Source: Adapted from *Depression in Late Life* (p. 24) by D. G. Blazer II, 1982, St. Louis, Mo.: C. V. Mosby. Copyright 1982 by C. V. Mosby. Adapted with permission.

The first part of an evaluation for depression consists of exploring current symptoms, feelings, and problems. Older persons should be allowed to tell their stories in their own words, proceeding at their own pace, if possible. Notes should be made of important points; specific questions can follow at an appropriate time later in the interview. It is important to remember that older persons will frequently not complain of depression or sadness, but will rather focus on physical complaints, worries, or family or financial problems. Careful observation and questioning will, however, usually uncover depressive symptoms. Inquiries should include questions as to both medical and psychiatric symptoms, their onset, frequency, duration, and recurrence.

Several themes frequently recur in the interviews of older people (Blazer, 1982). One common subject is that of physical complaints—aches, pains, insomnia, and the topic of medications. For the elderly, these subjects may arise, in part, due to the combination of increased bodily malfunction and decreased sphere of interests (Verwoerdt, 1976). In addition, the language of physical disabilities and medications is frequently for many elderly the verbal coin of exchange with friends and family. Another common theme is that of the past. Elders frequently spend a great deal of time reminiscing. This process of life review, as described by Butler (1963), includes reflections on aspects of prior events, successes, failures, and losses. Sharing such reminiscences with the elder can build rapport and uncover facts important to the assessment. Often, the older person speaks about fears, including those of losing physical and mental capacities, becoming a burden on loved ones, becoming financially destitute, and being institutionalized. Death is also a frequent topic for the elderly. Religious thoughts, discussion of funeral plans, and bequests are often part of the everyday conversation of older persons, both depressed and nondepressed.

What, then, are the symptoms of late-life depression for which the assessor should be alerted? Table 2–1 shows the most common symptoms and observable signs of depression in older persons. Table 2–2 compares symptoms commonly found in old age groups with those found more frequently among younger patients. The table includes symptoms that have been found in association with suicidality in old age as well as those that commonly occur in elders who have not been diagnosed with a depressive disorder.

Medical and Psychiatric History

Discussion of the past medical and psychiatric history often intermingles with that of the present in an interview with an older person. During the elder's recounting of the past, the examiner should give special attention to any prior psychiatric difficulties, including manic, depressive, or other symptoms, and to a history of medical problems, such as malignancy, infection, cardiovascular and endocrine (glandular) disease, disturbances of the senses, and neurological disease or deficits. Although evidence of causal relationships is still unclear, it is known that there is an increased association of depressive symptoms in the presence of these medical conditions, among others.

Table 2–3 outlines the differential diagnosis of elderly depression, including medical and psychiatric etiologies. As can be seen, substance-induced organic

Table 2–2 Elements of Depressive States Common to Older Versus Younger Age Groups

More Common to Older Age Group	More Common to Younger Age Group
• Decreased life satisfaction[a] Loss of interest	• Sadness, dejected mood
• Withdrawal from social environment[b]	• Use of term *depression* to identify feeling state
• Sense of emptiness[b]	• Feelings of guilt, self-blame
• Pessimism about future[a, b]	• Low self-esteem
• Cognitive symptoms (especially slowed thought, poor concentration)[a]	• Appetite loss
• Rumination over problems	• Suicidal thoughts, discussions
• Poor physical health[a, b]	• Suicidal gestures, incomplete attempts
• Recent bereavement[a, b]	• Use of suicide threat for manipulation
• Pseudodementia	
• Sleep difficulty,[a] if severe insomnia[b]	
• Somatic complaints (especially digestive, pain, cardiac)[a]	
• Hypochondria[b]	
• Agitation[b]	
• Weight loss	
• Loss of motivation	
• Vegetative signs (especially constipation)	
• Completed suicide	

[a] Also common in late life with depressive state.

[b] Associated with increased suicide risk in the elderly.

Source: Adapted from *Depression in Late Life* (p. 27) by D. G. Blazer II, 1982, St.Louis, Mo.: C. V. Mosby. Copyright 1982 by C. V. Mosby. Adapted with permission.

---

disorders feature prominently in the differential diagnosis of late-life depression. Thus, careful medication history should be taken, including both prescription and over-the-counter drugs. The latter should be pursued specifically, as many elderly do not regard such preparations as "drugs." Substance-induced depressive symptoms may be caused by one drug alone; more often, however, the symptoms are due to the additive effects of several medications, for example, the effects of mixing drugs and alcohol or of the combination of a powerful drug and the debilitated state of an elderly person. Medications for which to be especially alert include sleeping preparations,

Table 2-3 Differential Diagnosis of Depressive Signs and Symptoms
in the Elderly

   I. Organic mental disorders
     A. Dementias arising in the sensorium
       1. Primary degenerative dementia, senile onset, with depression
       2. Multiinfarct dementia
     B. Substance-induced organic mental disorder with depression
       1. Alcohol intoxication
       2. Barbiturates or similarly acting sedative or hypnotic intoxication
       3. Caffeine intoxication
       4. Antihypertensive agents, such as guanethedine and reserpine
       5. Antiarrhythmic agents such as propranolol
     C. Organic affective syndrome secondary to
       1. Hypothyroidism
       2. Cushing's syndrome
       3. Occult malignancy, such as carcinoma of the pancreas
       4. Vitamin deficiency syndromes, especially a deficiency in the B-complex
         vitamins and folic acid
       5. Mass lesions of the brain, especially slowly growing lesions affecting
         the frontal lobe, such as a meningioma

  II. Paranoid disorder: Individuals with paranoid disorders of late onset may demonstrate a significant depressive affect.

 III. Schizoaffective disorder: Uncommon in late life

 IV. Affective disorders
     A. Bipolar disorder
       1. Mixed
       2. Depressed
     B. Major depression
       1. Single-episode
       2. Recurrent
     C. Cyclothymic disorder
     D. Dysthymic disorder (or depressive neurosis)

   V. Anxiety disorders: Depressive symptoms are likely to accompany generalized anxiety disorders (anxiety neurosis) or obsessive-compulsive disorder (neurosis).

  VI. Somatoform disorder
     A. Psychogenic pain disorder
     B. Hypochondriasis (or hypochondriacal neurosis)

 VII. Adjustment disorder with depressed mood

VIII. Psychologic factors affecting physical conditions: One may see in the elderly a depressed affect associated with almost any acute or chronic physical illness.

  IX. Personality disorders: A depressed affect frequently accompanies narcissistic, dependent, and compulsive personality disorders in the elderly.

   X. Other
     A. Uncomplicated bereavement
     B. Marital problems
     C. Phases of a life problem or other life-circumstance problem
     D. Parent-child problem
     E. Other specified family circumstances
     F. Other interpersonal problems

  XI. Sleep disorders

"nerve pills" (including tranquilizers and other psychiatric drugs), digestive preparations, and cardiac and antihypertensive (blood pressure) medications. The use of habit-forming and recreational drugs, including tobacco, caffeine, and alcohol, should be explored. Excess caffeine, or caffeine intoxication, can cause symptoms of agitation, insomnia, and fears of mental deterioration in the elderly.

Alcohol continues to be the central nervous system drug most commonly used by the elderly. Although the association of alcohol abuse, depression, and suicidality appears high for every age group, it is known to be increased among the suicidal elderly (Blazer, 1982). Moreover, there is some evidence that pathologic drinking patterns can have their onset in later life. In a study by Schuckit and Miller (1976) of medical and psychiatric geriatric patients, one-half of the group with alcohol problems had onset of their drinking after age 41; many of this group had symptoms suggesting a depressive disorder.

An important part of evaluating any older person is an interview with the elder's family and/or supporting figures, including several generations, if possible. Depressive symptoms, such as agitation, apathy, or suspiciousness, may cause the elder's own rendition to be incomplete. Moreover, the family or others may be able to give a history of personality change even when the subject denies symptoms. The assessor should document any family history of psychiatric problems, including alcoholism and suicide, and of medical conditions associated with depression symptoms. It is especially important that the interviewer note the feelings evidenced between the elder and the elder's family and important others.

Physical Examination and Laboratory Tests

Although the relationship between physical and mental illness is, as noted, still unclear, it is evident that, because of an increased prevalence of physical illness and disability in the aged, the likelihood is increased that an elder with depressive symptoms will also have current or past medical problems. Studies such as that of Butler and Lewis (1977) have found that 86 percent of the depressed elderly have chronic health problems. When Schwab, Clemmons, Bialow, Duggan, and Davis (1965) studied medically ill patients, they found some depressive symptoms in all of them; indeed, in a group of hospitalized, medically ill patients, they found that 20 percent were clinically depressed. It is therefore evident that a thorough physical examination is an essential part of evaluating any elder. The examination should include a search for evidence of overt or covert medical illness, with special emphasis on those diseases with increased association to depression, as noted above. Assessors who are not trained to, or choose not to, perform the physical examination themselves should make the appropriate referral, being certain that the examination is completed and that further studies are undertaken as needed. Basic laboratory studies that should be done include a complete blood cell count, a urinalysis, and a determination of thyroxine level VDRL (serum test for syphilis). Studies that may be indicated as the evaluation proceeds include further medical and radiographic tests, an electroencephalogram, spinal fluid serology, computerized axial tomography, and vitamin B-12 and folate levels.

In addition to the laboratory determinations mentioned above, there are several neuroendocrinologic tests, recently emerged from research into clinical practice, that can aid the diagnosis of severe depression. The Dexamethasone Suppression Test (DST) involves testing the body's response to a synthetic steroid that, when taken by mouth, usually suppresses secretion of cortisol for up to 24 hours (Carroll et al., 1981). After baseline studies, the drug is given orally at 11 P.M.; the next day, two or three serial determinations are made of serum cortisol. Many studies have confirmed that up to 50 percent of seriously depressed patients will have test values elevated above the normal of 5 mcgms/ml. Moreover, successful somatic therapy of these same patients will usually result in a return of the test response to normal; thus both recovery and relapse can be monitored by following the DST. There has been some indication that the DST may be helpful in differentiating between depressed elderly patients who have pseudodementia (discussed later in this chapter) and those who have true dementia. Preliminary test results have been mixed; however, some authors feel that the test may be useful in distinguishing depression and dementia that is mild, but not severe (Jenike, 1983). The DST should be used in any elderly patient for whom the question of serious depression presents a diagnostic dilemma.

Two other psychoendocrinologic tests of research interest are now being used clinically. The TRH stimulation test involves testing the level of thyrotropin (TSH) secreted by the body in response to infusion of thyrotropin-releasing hormone (TRH). This response has been found to be blunted in 25 to 56 percent of patients with major depression and, in addition, is abnormal in some alcoholics, manics, and patients with anorexia nervosa (Loosen & Prange, 1982). Unlike the DST, the TRH test frequently does not normalize after successful treatment for major depression. An interesting speculation is that, while the DST may be a "state marker" (a characteristic that is an aspect of the illness itself, being present neither before nor after the illness), the TRH may actually be a "trait marker," which is present before, during, and after illness. If so, the TRH response may help in assessing a nondepressed subject's vulnerability to depressive illness (Loosen & Prange, 1982).

The combined use of DST and TRH tests may be diagnostically helpful, since there is evidence of no significant association between the two tests. Thus a person with major depression who is negative on the DST may well be positive on the TRH test, or vice versa. One recent study, involving 153 patients, found a sensitivity of 67 percent with combined use of the tests in identifying major depressives, as opposed to schizophrenics and nondepressed hospitalized patients. Furthermore, 82 percent of the DST-positive patients normalized at a time correlating significantly with clinical improvement. As expected, only 42 percent of TRH-positive patients normalized after successful treatment; however, none of these patients suffered a relapse within six months. In contrast, of the patients with persistent neuroendocrine abnormality, the majority in both groups did relapse; the use of prophylactic antidepressant medication did not avert relapse in nine of eleven relapsed patients who showed persistent neuroendocrine dysregulation (Targum, 1983). The GH test, a stimulation test similar to the TRH test, involves determining the secretory level of pituitary growth hormone (GH) in response to stimulation by various substances. More large-scale studies are needed, but present data in some studies suggest that up to 50 to 90 percent of major depressives may have a blunted GH response. However, as the response is also blunted in persons with many other diagnoses, some authors suggest that the GH test may best be used to help rule out a diagnosis of major depression (Carroll, 1980).

Another important new diagnostic study emerging from the research sector into clinical practice is the sleep electroencephalogram (EEG). Disruptions of the sleep-wake cycle, including sleep continuity, rapid eye movement (REM) activity, density and latency, are characteristic of several states, including normal old age, depression, and dementia. REM sleep is one of the elements of normal sleep, occurring several times during the night; it is characterized by a specific pattern on the sleep EEG. The period of REM latency is the amount of time that passes from the onset of sleep until the first REM period begins. In normal adults, REM latency is 60 minutes or more; however, it may be reduced to 30–50 minutes or less in persons suffering from major depressive illness (Coble, Kupfer & Shaw, 1981). In addition to increased REM activity and density, depressed subjects often have numerous waking periods. Recent studies have indicated that depressives show more disturbances on sleep EEG recordings than normals and that the severities of the disturbances and depression are positively correlated (Spiker, Coble, Cofsky, Foster, & Kupfer, 1980). Work by Coble et al. (1981) indicates that patients with extremely short REM latency (less than 10 minutes) may respond inadequately to tricyclic antidepressants only and may require treatment with combined pharmacotherapy or ECT to remit. Interestingly, similar patterns of disturbances are often seen in normal aging, depression, and dementia; however, one recent pilot study has demonstrated that elderly patients with dementia show significantly less sleep EEG disturbances than those with depression (Reynolds, Spiker, Hanin, & Kupfer, 1983). As more sleep laboratories are established in psychiatric diagnostic centers, the diagnostic sleep EEG will become an important tool for differential diagnosis of depressive symptoms in the elderly.

Mental Status Examination

An important part of assessing the elderly for depression consists of evaluating current mental function. Older persons, especially if depressed, may fluctuate a great deal in their mental abilities. Mental status should therefore be tested several times, preferably on different days and at different times of the day. Observations are carried out in several ways, including formal testing of abilities, questioning as to feelings and thoughts, and observing ~~ancillary~~ or nonverbal evidence of disordered mental function.

A mental status examination consists of evaluating the following:

- *Consciousness and orientation.* This area is evaluated by formal testing. It includes noting to what degree the subject is awake, alert, and aware of the surroundings. Does the subject know the day, the time of the day, and who and where the subject is? It is important to demand that the older person answer these questions in exact detail. Disorders of orientation are frequently missed because assessors assume that the cooperative, friendly elder is properly oriented (Wells & Duncan, 1980).
- *Mood and affect.* This area is evaluated by questioning and observation. Mood refers to a person's subjective feeling state; affect is the observed, objective evidence of that feeling state. Throughout the interview, the assessor should be aware of the older person's mood and affect, noting whether they fluctuate and if they are appropriate to verbal content. Both mood and affect may fluctuate less in the older depressive than in the younger.
- *Motor behavior.* The assessment of the motor abilities of the older person is frequently omitted, yet may provide evidence of neurological problems, as well as corroborative evidence of depressive illness. This area is evaluated by both formal testing and observation. To determine disorders of station, the subject is asked to stand, with feet together, with eyes open, then closed. Next, the subject is asked to stand on each foot, with eyes open. Gait is observed by watching the subject walk up a hall and return. Difficulties, ranging from clumsiness or limping to tremor and falling, should be recorded and evaluated further as necessary. The motor aspects of behavior, evaluated by observation and questioning, include psychomotor retardation or agitation. Depressed elderly may demonstrate any level of retardation, varying from none to slight slowing to profound apathy or catatonic stupor. However, severe depression in

the elderly frequently is manifested by agitated behaviors, as outlined in Table 2-1.

- *Perception.* Disorders in this area, evaluated by questioning and observation, include hallucinations and other distorted perceptions, such as those of time or distance. Elderly depressed patients do not commonly hallucinate; if present, their hallucinations usually involve auditory perceptions (such as hearing voices) and unusual bodily sensations or smells.

- *Thought processes and content.* This area is evaluated by questioning, observation, and occasionally by specific testing when defects are uncovered. The subject is observed for evidence of impaired ability to comprehend what is being said or to respond, either with words or actions, to what is being asked. Is there evidence or complaints that thought processes are slowed, speeded up, or confused? Are there obsessions, preoccupations, ruminations? In elderly patients, the theme of these preoccupations is often health, money matters, or domestic tasks; less often is it guilt and self-accusation, as in younger depressives. Does the subject speak of, or act as if the subject had, unusual beliefs or delusions that are not consistent with reality? Common delusions in severely depressed elders include those of being a victim of terminal illness, such as cancer; having vital organs that have died; having lost one's memory or mind; and of being useless. A deluded elder will be fixed in the belief, no matter what objective evidence there is to the contrary. Suicidal ideation may be part of the elder's thought content; this area requires careful evaluation and will be discussed in detail in other chapters.

- *Memory and intelligence.* This area is evaluated by observation, questioning, and formal testing. The assessment includes examination of immediate recall, recent memory, general fund of information, calculations, abstract thinking, problem solving, understanding, language abilities, and constructional abilities. For a detailed discussion of this examination, the reader is referred to *Neurology for Psychiatrists* by Wells and Duncan (1980). An excellent short-form mental status examination that tests orientation, memory, and intelligence is the Mini-Mental State Examination, devised by M.F. Folstein, S.E. Folstein, and McHugh (1975). A copy of this examination is included in Appendix 2-A and can easily be administered by a lay interviewer in 5–10 minutes. It is useful for periodic reevaluation of older persons and has been standardized in use on thousands of elderly subjects. The Mini-Mental State Examination tests for orientation, immediate recall, calculations, recent memory, language (including comprehension, reading, writing, and production), and constructional ability.

A difficult diagnostic problem frequently encountered by anyone evaluating a depressed older person is in evaluating the subject who appears to function poorly on a mental status examination. Are apparent disorientation, confusion, and poor intellectual function caused by organic brain disease or by severe depression? The latter clinical picture, often called pseudodementia, has been found to be common in the severely depressed elderly. Although its etiology is not entirely clear, the condition may be related to apathy, inattention, and distractibility, combined with decreased sensory and neurobiological adaptive abilities. Most certainly, its differentiation from true dementia is quite important, for unlike true dementia, pseudodementia usually clears with successful treatment of underlying depression.

Table 2–4 lists factors that may be helpful in differentiating dementia from pseudodementia. Careful, repetitive assessments, combined with psychological testing and clinical, laboratory, and neuroendocrine studies, will often make the diagnosis clear. However, the two conditions frequently coexist; depression is not uncommon in the demented elder. When there is any evidence of depressive illness in the presence of dementia, a trial of therapy is indicated.

Reassessing the Depressed Elder

After completing the initial assessment—including serial mental status evaluations and all indicated laboratory determinations—the trained assessor can make a "working diagnosis," using DSM III criteria. Multiple diagnoses should be made on various axes; the category for atypical or evolving diagnosis may be used. Older persons should be assessed frequently for changes in condition that would warrant new diagnostic procedures or alterations in therapy or environmental management. Areas that require special emphasis during reevaluation include medical and mental status, level of depressive symptoms, and suicide potential, which will be discussed in a subsequent chapter.

The first area in need of constant review is the elder's medical status. New or persistent medical symptoms and evidence of alcohol or drug misuse should be evaluated, not only because these factors may signal developing or worsening physical problems but also because of the previously noted associations between medical illness, drug abuses, depression, and suicide. The mental status of the older depressed person should also be reviewed frequently. This can be done skillfully, without formal testing, by inserting questions during the usual interview that test for orientation, recall, recent

Table 2–4 Characteristics Commonly Distinguishing Pseudodementia from Dementia

Pseudodementia	Dementia
Short duration of symptoms	Long duration of symptoms
Strong sense of distress	Often unconcerned
Many, detailed complaints of cognitive loss	Few, vague complaints of cognitive loss
Recent and remote memory loss are equal	Recent memory loss is worse than remote
Attention, concentration often good	Attention, concentration usually poor
Memory gaps common	Memory gaps unusual
"Don't know" answer common	"Near miss" answers common
Emphasizes disabilities, failures	Conceals disability, emphasizes accomplishments
Makes little effort to perform	Struggles to perform tasks
Does not try to keep up	Uses notes, calendars to keep up
Performance varied on similar tasks	Consistently poor performance on similar tasks
Pervasive affect change	Affect shallow, labile
Social skills lost early	Social skills retained
Orientation tests: "don't know"	Orientation tests: mistakes unusual or usual
Behavior incongruent with severity of cognitive problem	Behavior compatible with severity of cognitive problem
Symptoms not often worse at night	Symptoms often worse at night
Prior positive psychiatric history common	Prior positive psychiatric history not common

Source: Adapted from *Neurology for Psychiatrists* (p. 93) by C. E. Wells and G. W. Duncan, 1980, Philadelphia: F.A. Davis. Copyright 1980 by F.A. Davis. Adapted with permission.

---

memory, and general information, and by checking for signs of developing incapacities. If evidence or complaints of difficulties arise, or if the older person begins to dissemble and cover up incapacities, further evaluation and therapy should begin promptly.

Depression Rating Scales

The development or worsening of depressive symptoms in the elderly is serious, and may be life threatening. Symptom rating scales and checklists can be used in periodically assessing symptom severity in the elderly. Numerous scales have been developed to assess the many factors apparently involved in elderly depression. Of these, only three symptom rating scales are discussed here. More extensive information on various rating scales for depression is available in the rating scale review by Waskow and Parloff (1975), the test measurement manual by Hargreaves (1976), and the early clinical drug evaluation unit manual (Guy, 1976). However, it is important that the assessor be aware of both the strengths and weaknesses of rating scale evaluations.

One recent study has outlined the problems involved in the clinical use of rating scales. In reviewing the results of a recent community depression study, Boyd et al. (1982) found that one-third of the community subjects who had been diagnosed by clinical interview as having major depression were not detected by the rating scale used (the Center for Epidemiologic Studies-Depression (CES-D)). In analyzing this discrepancy, it was found that several of the subjects manifested clear clinical evidence of depressive symptoms that were not endorsed on the scale. In some cases, the subjects denied previously expressed symptomatology when filling out the checklist; in others, the depressed subjects were too slowed, apathetic, or confused to complete the scale accurately.

Based on these and other observations, the following caveats in using depression rating scales should be kept in mind. First, a personal interview assessment should always accompany the clinical use of a depression rating scale or checklist. In addition, such a scale is probably best used not as a self-administered but as an interviewer-administered instrument. The interviewer should first read the scale items to the subject and then record the subject's responses. Finally, the best method of use may be to administer the checklist first and then proceed to the interview. In the clinical setting, this may be done by following the checklist administration with a discussion about its items, thereby eliciting more information about positive symptoms and reconfirming that the symptoms denied are indeed absent. Used in this way, scales or checklists may be a helpful means of assessing and following the older person's symptoms from interview to interview. In addition, since scales and checklists frequently detect high levels of symptoms in persons who are not clinically diagnosable as depressed (such as those suffering from acute adjustment reactions, recent bereavement, or medical illnesses causing depressive symptoms), they are useful in following the depressive symptoms of subjects who do not have diagnosed major or minor depressive disorders but who are both suffering and at risk for a major depression or suicidal ideation.

Three well-known and commonly used rating scales for depression are described below. A copy of one of these scales is included in Appendix 3-A.

Although these scales have often been used on elderly subjects, further research is needed on their validity and reliability in older populations.

The Hamilton Rating Scale (Hamilton, 1960) was devised in the late 1950s. It was designed to be used on persons already diagnosed as having a depressive disorder. Its purpose is to quantify the results of a clinical interview; therefore, interviewer skill is a crucial factor in its optimal use. Also, if more than one clinician uses the scale in a study, reliability can become a major issue. It is recommended that two raters initially score at the same interview independently. With practice, interrater correlation can be built to 0.90 (Hamilton, 1960). The scale contains 17 variables, several of which are rated as to intensity. In addition, four nonscored variables can be noted. Scores are summed for a final score. The Hamilton scale has the advantage of having become a standard measure that has been included in many clinical studies of depression. The following cutoff points have been standardized for depressive severity: less than 6, no depression; 17 or greater, mild depression; 24 to 25 or greater, severe depression.

In 1964, Zung developed a shorter scale, designed to be self-administered, for use in initial evaluation and follow-up reevaluation of depressed subjects (Zung, 1965). The Zung Self-Rating Depression Scale (SDS) (See Appendix 3-A) consists of 20 items, 10 using symptomatically positive wording and 10 symptomatically negative. The index for the SDS is derived by dividing the raw score by the maximal possible score of 80 (in the resulting score the decimal is dropped). The time period covered is the two weeks just prior to administration. The following are suggested guidelines for interpretation of the data: below 50, no significant depression; 50–59, minimal to mild depression; 60–69, moderate to marked depression; 70 and over, severe depression. The SDS has been translated into many languages and is widely used in international studies. Okimoto et al. (1982) have evaluated the SDS on 55 older persons, comparing ratings to clinical assessments made by psychiatrists blind to the rating scores. In 80 percent of the subjects, the SDS rating correlated with that of the interviewer (Okimoto et al., 1982). Another group, Steuer, Bank, Olsen, and Jarvik (1980), evaluated whether poor physical health in an elderly person could influence SDS ratings. They concluded that health is not a confounding factor in SDS ratings of older persons (Steuer et al., 1980).

The CES-D was developed in the mid-1970s by the Center for Epidemiologic Studies, arising from the need for a short, easily administered self-report of depressive symptoms for use in studying the epidemiology of psychiatric illness in a community. The items were derived from other, previously validated depression scales (Weissman, Sholomskas, Pottenger, Prusoff, & Locke, 1977). The scale consists of 20 items that assess symptoms for the week just prior to the interview. Each item is scored on a range of 0 to 4, with higher scores indicating more impairment, except on four items (Numbers 4, 8, 12, and 16) for which scoring is reversed. The total, summed score ranges from 0 to 60. The most widely used cutoff point for cases of depression is a score of 16 (Jenike, 1983). The scale is simple, easy to administer, and has been widely used in community populations. However, further evaluation of its use in elderly populations is desirable.

REFERENCES

American Psychiatric Association. (1980). *Diagnostic and statistical manual of mental disorders* (3rd ed.). Washington, D.C.: Author.

Beck, T. (1967). *Depression: Causes and treatment.* Philadelphia, Pa.: University of Pennsylvania Press.

Bibring, E. (1953). The mechanism of depression. In P. Greenacre (Ed.), *Affective disorders: Psychoanalytic contribution to their study* (pp. 13–48). New York: International Universities Press.

Blau, D. (1980, October). *Depression in late life: Psychodynamic aspects.* Paper presented at a conference on depression in late life, Cleveland, Ohio.

Blau, D., & Berezin, M. (1975). Neuroses and character disorders. In J. Howells (Ed.), *Modern perspectives in the psychiatry of old age* (pp. 201–233). New York: Brunner & Mazel.

Blazer, D. (1982). *Depression in late life.* St. Louis, Mo.: C. V. Mosby.

Boyd, J. H., Weissman, M. M., Thompson, D., & Myers, J. K. (1982). Screening for depression in a community sample. *Archives of General Psychiatry, 39,* 1195–1200.

Brown, B. L., Goodwin, F. K., Ballenger, J. C., Goyer, P. F., & Major, L. F. (1979). Aggression in humans correlates with cerebrospinal fluid amine metabolites. *Psychiatry Research, 1,* 131–139.

Butler, R. (1963). The life review: An interpretation of reminiscence in the aged. *Psychiatry, 26,* 65.

Butler, R. & Lewis, M. (1977). *Aging and mental health: Positive psychosocial approaches* (2nd Ed.). St. Louis, MO: C. V. Mosby.

Carroll, B. J. (1980). Implication of biological research for the diagnosis of depression. *Excerpta Medica, International Congress Series,* No. 531, 85–107.

Carroll, B. J., Feinburg, M., Greden, J. F., Tarika, J., Albala, A. A., Haskett, R. F., James, N. M., Kronfol, Z., Lohr, N., Steiner, M., de Vigne, J. P., & Young, E. (1981). A specific laboratory test for the diagnosis of melancholia: Standardization, validation and clinical utility. *Archives of General Psychiatry, 30,* 15–22.

Cath, S. (1965). Discussion notes. In M. Beregin & S. Cath (Eds.), *Geriatric psychiatry: Grief, loss and emotional disorder in the aging process* (pp. 128–129). New York: International Universities Press.

Coble, P. A., Kupfer, D. J., & Shaw, D. H. (1981). Distribution of REM latency in depression. *Biological Psychiatry, 16,* 453–446.

Dorland's illustrated medical dictionary (25th Ed.). Philadelphia: W. B. Saunders.

Erikson, E. (1959). Identity and the life cycle. In S. G. Klein (Ed.), *Psychological Issues* (Vol. 1, No. 1, p. 98). New York: International Universities Press.

Folstein, M. F., Folstein, S. E., & McHugh, P. R. (1975). "Mini-Mental State": A practical method for grading the cognitive state of patients for the clinician. *Journal of Psychiatric Research, 12,* 189–198.

Freud, S. (1924). Mourning and Melancholia. In *Sigmund Freud's Collected Papers* (Vol. 4, pp. 255–268). London: Hogarth Press.

Freud, S. (1957). Mourning and melancholia. In J. Streachey (Ed. and Trans.), *The standard edition of the complete psychological works of Sigmund Freud* (Vol. 14, pp. 237–258). London: Hogarth Press.

Guy, W. (Ed.). (1976). *ECDEU assessment manual for psychopharmacology* (No. ADM 76–336). Rockville, Md.: U. S. Department of Health, Education, and Welfare.

Hamilton, M. (1960). A rating scale for depression. *Journal of Neurology, Neurosurgery, and Psychiatry, 23,* 56–62.

Hargreaves, W. A. (1976). *Resource materials for community mental health program evaluation.* Rockville, Md.: U. S. Department of Health, Education, and Welfare.

Hartmann, E. (1973). *The functions of sleep.* New Haven, Conn.: Yale University Press.

Jenike, M. A. (1983). Dexamethasone suppression test as a clinical aid in elderly depressed patients. *Journal of American Geriatrics Society, 31,* 45–48.

Klein, M. (1948). *Contributions to psychoanalysis 1921-1945.* London: Hogarth Press.

Levine, S. (1965). Depression in the aged. In M. Berezin & S. Cath (Eds.), *Geriatric psychiatry: Grief, loss, and emotional disorder in the aging process* (pp. 210–216). New York: International Universities Press.

Loosen, P. T., & Prange, A. J. (1982). Serum thyrotropin response to thyrotropin-releasing hormones in psychiatric patients: A review. *American Journal of Psychiatry, 139,* 40.

McCarley, R., & Hobson, J. (1977). The neurobiological origins of psychoanalytic dream theory. *American Journal of Psychiatry, 134,* 1211–1221.

Okimoto, J. T., Barnes, R. F., Veith, R. C., Raskind, M. A., Inui, T. S., & Carter, W. B. (1982). Screening for depression in geriatric medical patients. *American Journal of Psychiatry, 239,* 799–802.

Reynolds, G. F., III, Spiker, D. G., Hanin, I., & Kupfer, D. J. (1983). Electroencephalographic sleep, aging and psychopathology: New data and state of the art. *Biological Psychiatry, 18,* 139–155.

Schildkraut, J. (1965). The catecholamine hypothesis of affective disorders: A review of supporting evidence. *American Journal of Psychiatry, 122,* 509.

Schuckit, M., & Miller, E. (1976). Alcoholism in elderly men: A survey of a general medical ward. *Annals of the New York Academy of Science, 273,* 558.

Schwab, J. J., Clemmons, R. S., Bialow, M., Duggan, V., & Davis, B. (1965). A study of the somatic symptomatology of depression in medical inpatients. *Psychosomatics, 6,* 273.

Spiker, D. G., Coble, P., Cofsky, J., Foster, F. G., & Kupfer, D. J. (1978). EEG sleep and severity of depression. *Biological Psychiatry, 13,* 485–488.

Spitz, R. (1946). Anaclitic depression. *Psychoanalytic Study of the Child, 2,* 313.

Steuer, J., Bank, L., Olsen, E. J., & Jarvik, L. F. (1980). Depression, physical health and somatic complaints in the elderly: A study of the Zung Self-Rating Depression Scale. *Journal of Gerontology, 35,* 683–688.

Targum, S. D. (1983). The application of serial neuroendocrine challenge studies in the management of depressive disorders. *Biological Psychiatry, 18,* 319.

Van Praag, H. (1982). Biochemical psychopathological predictors of suicidality. *Biblitheca Psychiatrica, 162,* 42–60.

Verwoerdt, A. (1976). *Clinical geropsychiatry.* Baltimore, Md.: Williams & Wilkins.

Waskow, I. G., & Parloff, M. B. (1975). *Psychotherapy change measures, report on the clinical research branch* (NIMH outcome measures project). Rockville, Md.: National Institute of Mental Health.

Weissman, M. M., Sholomskas, M., Pottenger, M., Prusoff, B. A., & Locke, B. Z. (1977). Assessing depressive symptoms in five psychiatric populations: A validation study. *American Journal of Epidemiology, 106,* 203–214.

Wells, C. E., & Duncan, G. W. (1980). *Neurology for psychiatrists.* Philadelphia: F. A. Davis.

Zetzel, E. (1965). Dynamics of the metapsychology of the aging process. In M. Berezin, & S. Cath (Eds.), *Geriatric psychiatry: Grief, loss, and emotional disorder in the aging process* (pp. 109–119). New York: International Universities Press.

Zung, W. K. (1965). A self-rating depression scale. *Archives of General Psychiatry, 12,* 63–70.

Appendix 2-A

Mini-Mental State Examination

Maximum
Score   *Score*

Orientation

5   ( ) What is the (year) (season) (date) (day) (month)?

5   ( ) Where are we: (state) (county) (town) (hospital) (floor)?

Registration

3   ( ) Name three objects: one second to say each. Then ask the patient all three after you have said them. Give one point for each correct answer. Then repeat them until the patient learns all three. Count trials and record.

Trials

Attention and Calculation

5   ( ) Serial 7s. One point for each correct. Stop after five answers. Alternatively, spell "world" backwards.

Recall

3   ( ) Ask for the three objects repeated above. Give 1 point for each correct answer.

Language

9   ( ) Name a pencil, and a watch (two points)
Repeat the following: "No ifs, ands or buts." (one point)
Follow a three-stage command: "Take a paper in your right hand, fold it in half, and put it on the floor" (three points)
Read and obey the following:

Close your eyes (one point)

Write a sentence (one point)
Copy design (one point)

Total score

Assess level of consciousness along a
continuum _____

        Alert   Drowsy   Stupor   Coma

Reprinted with permission from "Mini-Mental State: A Practical Method for Grading the Cognitive States of Patients for the Clinician" by M. F. Folstein, S. E. Folstein, and P. R. McHugh, 1975, *Journal of Psychiatric Research*, 12, pp.196–197. Copyright 1975 by Pergamon Press, Ltd.

Instructions for Administration of Mini-Mental State Examination

Orientation:

Ask for the date. Then ask specifically for parts omitted, e.g., "Can you also tell me what season it is?" One point for each correct answer.

Ask in turn, "Can you tell me the name of this hospital?" (town, county, etc.). One point for each correct answer.

Registration:

Ask the patient if you may test for memory. Then say the names of three unrelated objects, clearly and slowly, about one second for each. After you have said all three, ask the patient to repeat them. This first repetition determines the patient's score (0–3); but keep saying them until the patient can repeat all three, up to six trials. If the patient does not eventually learn all three, recall cannot be meaningfully tested.

Attention and Calculation:

Ask the patient to begin with 100 and count backwards by 7. Stop after five subtractions (93, 86, 79, 72, 65). Score the total number of correct answers.

If the patient cannot or will not perform this task, ask the patient to spell the word "world" backwards. The score is the number of letters in correct order. For example, dlrow = 5, dlorw = 3.

Recall:

Ask the patient to recall the three words you previously asked the patient to remember. Score 0–3.

Language:

Naming: Show a wrist watch and ask the patient what it is. Repeat for pencil. Score 0–2.

Repetition: Ask the patient to repeat the sentence after you. Allow only one trial. Score 0 or 1.

Three-stage command: Give the patient a piece of plain blank paper and repeat the command. Score one point for each part correctly executed.

Reading: On a blank piece of paper print the sentence, "Close your eyes," in letters large enough for the patient to see clearly. Ask the patient to read it and do what it says. Score one point only if the patient actually closes eyes.

Writing: Give the patient a blank piece of paper and ask the patient to write a sentence for you. Do not dictate the sentence; it is to be written spontaneously. It must contain a subject and verb and be sensible. Correct grammar and punctuation are necessary.

Copying: On a clean piece of paper, draw intersecting pentagons, each side about 1 in., and ask the patient to copy it exactly as it is. All ten angles must be presented and two must intersect to score one point. Tremor and rotation are ignored.

Estimate the patient's level of sensorium along a continuum, from alert on the left to coma on the right.

Chapter 3

Assessment of Personal Well-Being in the Elderly

In an early article, Robert Havighurst (1961) opened with this remark: "The science of gerontology has the practical purpose, we often say, of 'adding life to the years' of the latter part of the human lifespan. By 'adding life to the years' we mean helping people to enjoy life, and to get satisfaction from life" (p. 8). To measure successful aging we must know how much satisfaction an individual derives from life, and we should be able to assess subjective psychological well-being and personal happiness.

In this chapter, our concern is with the measurement of life satisfaction or morale, loneliness, and stress in the elderly. A close relationship has been established between psychological well-being and depression and between loneliness and depression. The accurate assessment of inner states of psychological well-being, such as morale and loneliness, is another important method of tapping emotional states in the elderly and of identifying those who are vulnerable to suicide. The various published measures of life satisfaction or morale, loneliness, and stress discussed in the following pages can be found in the appendix.

LIFE SATISFACTION OR MORALE

Since its beginning, a major concern in the gerontology field has been the measurement of psychological well-being, one indicator of "successful aging." Several definitions and conceptualizations of well-being have been developed over the years. The most frequently used are morale, life satisfaction, and adjustment. Such concepts imply happiness as a major factor in well-being; all of the instruments developed to measure well-being include items to tap personal happiness. To measure psychological well-being, various morale scales, life satisfaction indexes, and attitude scales have been developed to operationally define "successful aging." All such scales focus upon the

38

assessment of inner states of older individuals; they assume that older persons themselves know best how they feel and can best assess their own psychological well-being and happiness.

Morale scales or life satisfaction indexes for use with aged individuals can be used in conjunction with various depression measures to assess more accurately the emotional state of a particular older person. The validity of existing self-report measures of depression with elderly subjects has recently been questioned by several studies that indicate that the pattern of response to such measures by elderly subjects is distorted by the overlap between typical depressive symptomatology and changes associated with the aging process itself. They also suggest that age produces a differential pattern of response to such questionnaires, with the somatic symptoms being preferentially responded to, while emotional-psychological symptoms are under-reported (Oltman, Michals, & Steer, 1980; Schwab , Holzer, & Warheit, 1973; Zemore & Eames, 1979).

In spite of the fact that depression is the most common psychiatric disorder of the elderly and also one of the conditions most frequently misdiagnosed or missed, little interest has been shown by clinicians and other caregivers in utilizing existing instruments to evaluate emotional states in the elderly. In a recent review of the field, Janke and Baltisson (1979) noted that the principal measures of such states, developed specifically with the aged, have been life-satisfaction or morale questionnaires that, although they purport to measure stable traits or attitudes, actually fairly accurately reflect mood. Morris, Wolf, and Klerman (1975) administered the Philadelphia Geriatric Center Morale Scale, a fairly well-known measure of morale, and the Zung Self-Rating Depression Scale (See Appendix 3-A) to 120 state hospital patients with a mean age of 53. They found considerable conceptual and informational overlap between the two. Analysis revealed that several items on both scales distinguished clinical depression and were mathematically similar. Specifically, they discovered considerable common variance between the mood and morale scales. Wilmott and Vaddadi (1981) also found that life satisfaction measures developed for use with an elderly population effectively distinguished between groups of clinically depressed elderly and "normals"; the measures were also differentially sensitive to the effects of change in clinical state.

Such findings demonstrate the existence of a common theme across independently constructed scales of depression and morale and suggest that depression and low morale or life satisfaction are, to some degree, equivalent moods. In other words, it is possible that life satisfaction or morale questionnaires can function independently, and just as effectively, as standard self-report mood questionnaires in evaluating emotional disorders and identifying vulnerability in the elderly. Life satisfaction or morale measures may reflect depression as a persistent trait rather than as a temporary state. Demoralization syndromes are measured by the Life Satisfaction Index A or B, the Philadelphia Geriatric Center Morale Scale, and other similar instruments that tap attitudes toward the quality of past, present, and future phases of life. (See Appendix 3-B.)

The first measure of well-being was developed in 1949 by Cavan, Burgess, Havighurst, and Goldhammer (1949). Their Attitude Inventory, also called the Cavan Scale (see Appendix 3-B), was developed to measure personal adjustment to aging. They defined adjustment as "the individual's restructuring of his attitudes and behavior in such a way as to integrate the expression of his aspiration with the expectations and demands of his society" (p. 10). The Cavan scale takes into account a person's association with family, friends, and formal and informal groups, as well as the person's feelings of importance and satisfaction with these activities and statuses. The scale consists of eight components (health, friendship, family, work, finances, religion, usefulness, and happiness) with seven questions about each. The 56 items all have the same response format: agree, disagree, or uncertain. The instrument can be administered orally or in written form. The score is computed by taking the sum of the agree answers to the positive items (in each of the eight components, three items are stated positively) minus the sum of the agree answers to the negative items (three items in each of the eight components are stated negatively), yielding a total score of -24 to +24. Cavan and her associates reported a test-retest correlation of .72 based on 110 persons and a split-half reliability estimate of .95 based on 200 persons. In a test of validity, they reported a correlation of .74 between the ratings of independent judges and reports of interviewers. In another test, Havighurst (1951) reported correlations of .73 between the scale and interviewers' ratings of adjustment.

The earliest scale developed to measure morale equates morale with adjustment. The Kutner Morale Scale (see Appendix 3-B) developed by Kutner, Fanshel , Togo, and Langner, was used in their well-known study (1956) of the elderly in the Kips Bay Area of New York. They defined morale as "a continuum of responses to life and living problems that reflect the presence or absence of satisfaction, optimism, and expanding life perspectives" (p. 48). Their scale is a unidimensional measure of morale consisting of seven Guttman-type items, such as, "All in all, how much unhappiness would you say you find in life today?" A value of 1 is assigned to each correct response to the seven items, as determined by a trained interviewer who administers the scale orally. Scores can range from a low of 0 to a high of 7. The coefficient of reproducibility of the seven items as a whole is 90 percent (Kutner et al., 1956). In a formal test of validity of this scale, Lohmann

(1977) reported correlations with nine other measures of well-being ranging from .397 to .883. (See Appendix 3-B.)

Another major measure of morale has been developed more recently by M. Powell Lawton for use with those aged 70 and over. The Philadelphia Geriatric Center Morale Scale (PGC) (see Appendix 3-B), developed in 1972 and revised in 1975, is an attempt to measure morale in a multidimensional manner. Morale, as defined by Lawton, implies a basic sense of satisfaction with oneself, a feeling that there is a place for oneself in the environment, and an acceptance of what cannot be changed (Lawton, 1972). When subjected to a principal-component analysis, the original 22-item scale yielded six factors: (1) Attitude Toward Own Aging—items that measure self-perceived change as one ages and self-evaluation of the quality of these changes; (2) Agitation—items relating to anxiety and dysphoric mood; (3) Loneliness Dissatisfaction—items that reflect the extent to which an individual feels lonely and dissatisfied with life; (4) Acceptance of Status Quo—items measuring general satisfaction with the way things are; (5) Optimism—items that relate to the capacity to enjoy immediate pleasures; and (6) Surgency—items that reflect an optimistic outlook and ideology, a readiness to remain active, and freedom from anxiety (Lawton, 1975). After a series of factor analyses on the original scale conducted by Lawton (1975) and Morris and Sherwood (1975) on new and larger samples of elderly, the scale was revised into a 17-item scale comprising only three components: Attitude Toward Own Aging, Agitation, and Lonely Dissatisfaction. The 17 items generally require a yes or no response; they can be responded to orally or in written form. Each high-morale response scores as 1; the points are then summed for a total morale score ranging from 1 to 17. The following are sample items: "I sometimes worry so much that I can't sleep" (Agitation). "As you get older you are less useful" (Attitude Toward Own Aging). "I see enough of my family and friends" (Lonely Dissatisfaction). The three factors on the revised 17-item scale have a high degree of internal consistency: .85, .81, and .85. In his validation studies, Lawton found a correlation of .47 between morale scores and judges' rankings for a sample of institutionalized elderly (N = 199). A later study of validity by Lohmann found the correlation between the morale scale and the Life Satisfaction Index A to be .76 (George & Bearon, 1980).

Happiness has been measured most directly by the Bradburn Affect-Balance Scale (Bradburn, 1969). (See Appendix 3-B.) This scale can be used with a variety of age groups. Happiness is measured as the difference between positive and negative affect expressed by the respondent. The 10-item scale consists of five items that measure positive affect and five that measure negative affect. For example, the respondent is asked, "During the past few weeks did you ever feel pleased (or bored) about having accomplished something?" The scale may be given orally or in written form. To score the scale, each yes response to an item is given a score of 1. The responses are then summed separately for the five items that reflect positive affect and for the five items that reflect negative affect. The difference between the scores on the positive and negative items is then computed, resulting in a score range from –5 to +5. Graney (1975) and Mangen (1977) have shown that the scale can effectively measure happiness in an elderly population. Bradburn (1969) reported test-retest reliability values (N = 200) of a .86 to .96 for positive-affect items and .90 to .97 for negative-affect items. Mangen (1977) reported internal consistency estimates, using Cronbach's alpha, of .66 for positive affect and .70 for negative affect for the National Council on the Aging (NCOA) (1975) study on aging in America. In a test of validity, Moriwaki (1974) reported that the Affect-Balance Scale is positively correlated with morale (r = .61).

The first index of life satisfaction, the Life Satisfaction Index (LSI), was developed by Neugarten, Havighurst, and Tobin (1961). (See Appendix 3-B.) This index has two forms: the Life Satisfaction Index A (LSI-A) and the Life Satisfaction Index B (LSI-B). More recently, Lohmann (1977) has proposed a different Life Satisfaction Index.

The LSI has five components of life satisfaction, each component comprising five items scored from 1 to 5: (1) Zest versus Apathy—items that measure the extent to which the person takes pleasure from life's daily activities and from people and things; (2) Resolution and Fortitude—items that measure the extent to which an individual regards life as meaningful and resolutely accepts that which life has offered; (3) Congruence Between Desired and Achieved Goals—items that tap the degree to which a person feels major life goals have been achieved; (4) Positive Self-Concept—items that reflect whether or not an individual has a positive self-image; and (5) Mood Tone—items that measure the degree to which one maintains happy and optimistic attitudes and moods (Neugarten et al., 1961). The LSI-A, usually administered in written form, contains 20 statements with which the person can agree or disagree. The LSI-B consists of 12 items (6 open-ended and 5 checklist-type) with two or three response categories for each. Scoring of both the LSI-A and LSI-B is done by summing correct responses. Scores on the LSI-A range from a low of 0 to a high of 20. Scores on the LSI-B range from a low of 0 to a high of 23.

Adams (1969) examined the reliability of the LSI-A and reported that all items except Item 11 fell within the acceptable range of 20 to 80 percent. More recently, Knapp (1977) reported validity coefficients of .55 and .39 with the ratings of lay interviewers and clinical psychologists, respectively, for the LSI-A. Neugarten et al. (1961) found a correlation of .55 for the LSI-A and the original Life Satisfaction Index and a correlation of .58 for the LSI-B and the LSI. Lohmann (1977) reported correlations of the LSI-A and LSI-B with nine other measures of psychological well-being ranging from .385 to .883.

Based upon factor analyses of 10 measures of psychological well-being administered to 259 people aged 60 and over, Lohmann (1977) developed a Life Satisfaction Scale consisting of 18 closed-end items to which a person can agree or disagree. The scale borrows items from six other existing scales. Sample items include, "I feel just miserable most of the time," "I have a lot to be sad about," "These are the best years of my life." Lohmann reports a reliability coefficient of .88 (Lohmann, 1977).

LONELINESS

Definitions

Loneliness has been variously defined in the literature. In their comprehensive sourcebook on the subject, Peplau and Perlman (1982) cite the following definitions:

> I define loneliness as the absence or perceived absence of satisfying social relations, accompanied by symptoms of psychological distress that are related to the actual or perceived absence.... *I propose that social relationships can be treated as a particular class of reinforcement....* [emphasis added] Therefore, loneliness can be viewed in part as a response to the absence of important social reinforcements. (Young, 1982, p. 380)

> Loneliness is caused not by being alone but by being without some definite needed relationship or set of relationships. Loneliness appears always to be a response to the absence of some particular type of relationship or, more accurately, a response to the absence of some particular relational provision. (Weiss, 1973, p. 17)

> Loneliness ... is the exceedingly unpleasant and driving experience connected with inadequate discharge of the need for human intimacy, for interpersonal intimacy. (Sullivan, 1953, p. 290)

> Loneliness ... is an experienced discrepancy between the kinds of interpersonal relationships the individual perceives himself as having at the time, and the kinds of relationships he would like to have, either in terms of his past experience or some ideal state that he has actually never experienced. (Sermat, 1978, p. 274)

> Loneliness . . . refers to an affective state in which the individual is aware of the feeling of being apart from others, along with the experience of a vague need for other individuals. (Leiderman, 1980, p. 387)

> In our view, loneliness is caused by the absence of an appropriate social partner who could assist in achieving important other-contingent goals, and the continuing desire for such social contacts. (Derlega & Margulis, 1982, p. 155)

In his well-known relational-deficit typology of loneliness, Weiss (1973) makes a distinction between the loneliness of "emotional isolation" and the loneliness of "social isolation." Loneliness of emotional isolation appears in the absence of a close emotional attachment and results in feelings of emptiness; whereas loneliness of social isolation is associated with the absence of an engaging social network, resulting in feelings of boredom, rejection, and marginality. Moustakas (1972) similarly distinguishes two kinds of loneliness, "non-being" and "cut-offness," corresponding to Weiss' loneliness of emotional isolation and loneliness of social isolation.

However scholars may differ in the details of their definitions, there appear to be three important points of agreement in the ways they view loneliness (Peplau & Perlman, 1982): (1) Loneliness results from deficiencies in a person's social relationships. (2) Loneliness is a subjective experience and is not synonymous with objective social isolation; people can be alone without being lonely. (3) The experience of loneliness is unpleasant and distressing. An important common element in most definitions of loneliness is that the aloneness or isolation being experienced is emotionally distressing. Loneliness may be transient, situational, or chronic (lasting two years or longer).

Psychological Concepts

There are three main approaches to conceptualizing the psychological foundations of loneliness:

1. The first approach emphasizes cognitive processes concerning people's perception and evaluation of their social relations. The emphasis here is on the subjective evaluation of social relationships as fulfilling the need for social interaction, both quantitatively and qualitatively, to the person's satisfaction (Flanders, 1976). Peplau and Perlman (1982) suggest that each person has an optimal level of social interaction. When social relations are suboptimal, a person experiences the distress of loneliness; on the

other hand, excessive social contact may produce a feeling of "crowding" and social stimulus overload.

2. A second approach suggests that the main deficiency experienced by lonely people is insufficient "social reinforcement." Social relations are seen as a special class of reinforcement. Dependent on past reinforcement history, a person finds a specific quantity and type of social relationship satisfying. High past satisfaction in social relationships might incline one to feel more pain in deficit or loss of social interaction than if one had not experienced such positive reinforcement (Young, 1982).

3. The third approach emphasizes inherent human needs for intimacy, relatedness, or "homonymy." Theorists advocating this approach claim that social relationships are a basic need of humans. Loneliness is the feeling that arises when the nature of social stimuli fails to satisfy qualitatively and quantitatively the basic need for intimacy, acceptance, and love. Because this need is so basic and obviously felt, the cognitive process emphasis on perceptual dissatisfaction is reflected in human behavior, beginning with the infant's crying, which can only be stopped by picking up and cuddling the infant, and extending to the self-destruction of an old person who can no longer stand the pain of loneliness. Also, since social relationships are so basic a need, the presence or absence of social reinforcement (the presence or absence of social relationships that are both qualitatively and quantitatively satisfying) becomes a potent source of pleasure or pain. Thus, it would seem that the most complete treatment of loneliness must be grounded on the universal need of intimacy from infancy throughout life, demonstrated by activity (social reinforcement) meeting the need, with a resulting cognitively affective state of satisfaction or distress. In short, the satisfaction of the need for intimacy and social interaction furnishes humans' greatest satisfaction with love and joy. Conversely, a severe deficit in social relationships—a lack of love or loss of intimacy—brings humans the greatest stress and deepest psychic pain, experienced as loneliness.

At this point, we should note two major differences between the social needs and cognitive theories. The affective aspects of loneliness are emphasized by the social needs approach, while the cognitive approach centers on the perception and evaluation of social relations and relational deficits. A second difference is in the degree of necessary self-perception. The needs approach suggests that people may experience loneliness without explicitly defining themselves as lonely. In contrast, the cognitive theorists feel that they must work with those who perceive themselves as lonely and report relational inadequacies.

Artists, poets, novelists, and songwriters have all commented on the agony, anguish, emptiness, and fear of loneliness. Loneliness is a negative emotional state that implies alienation, lack of close emotional ties, suboptimal social interaction and reinforcement, and feelings of rejection, isolation, and marginality. In describing the emotional state of loneliness, Sadler & Johnson (1980) note that it is a condition in which "we feel left out, cut off, lost, forgotten, unwanted, unneeded, and ignored" (p. 38).

Hyams (1969) has noted that loneliness can profoundly aggravate the emotional components of an illness by producing feelings of insecurity and, later, possibly apathy. Similarly, David Riesman wrote, "So great is the shame of the lonely, they withdraw further out of fear of additional experience of loss" (Burnside, 1980, p. 731).

Like depression, loneliness is filled with helplessness, pessimism, and pain. Fromm-Reichman (1959) has suggested that severe loneliness is character- ized by "paralyzing hopelessness and unutterable futility" (p. 7); and Weiss (1973) has characterized loneliness as a "gnawing distress without redeeming features" (p. 15).

For Gregory Zilboorg (1938), one of the first psychodynamically oriented psychiatrists to deal with the topic of loneliness, the psychodynamics of loneliness are similar to, if not identical to, the psychodynamics of depression. Very often, loneliness precedes and precipitates depression; seldom does one encounter a severe depression without a critical component of loneliness. Whether one regards loneliness as a subset of depression or as a separate clinical entity, there is substantial overlap between loneliness and depression. Research has shown correlations between loneliness and depression ranging from .38 (Russell, Peplau, & Ferguson, 1978) to .71 (Young, 1979b) depending on the populations examined and the instruments used.

A review of the literature reveals that loneliness is consistently linked with depression (Bragg, 1979; Russell, Peplau, & Cutrona, 1980; Schultz & Moore, 1982; Weeks, Michela, Peplau, & Bragg, 1980; Young, 1982). Loneliness has been found to be positively associated with feelings of low self-esteem (Jones, 1982; Loucks, 1980; Wood, 1978), unhappiness and pessimism (Bradburn, 1969; Perlman, Gerson, & Spinner, 1978), and self-consciousness (Jones, Freeman, & Goswick, 1981). It has also been linked with somatic complaints (Berg, Melstrom, Persson, & Svanborg, 1981; Kivett, 1979), physical health problems (Siegler, Nowlin, & Blumenthal, 1980), and suicide (Wenz, 1977).

In their comprehensive study, Rubenstein and Shaver (1982) identified through factor analysis four feeling states most frequently associated with loneliness: Desperation (desperate, panicked, helpless, afraid, abandoned, without hope, vulnerable); Depression (sad, depressed, empty, isolated, sorry for self, melancholy, alienated, longing to be with one special person); Impatient Boredom (impatient, bored, desire to be elsewhere, uneasy, angry, unable to concentrate); and Self-Depreciation (unattractive, down on self, stupid, ashamed, insecure). In other words, those who scored highest on the loneliness scale used by Rubenstein and Shaver also demonstrated significantly more often feelings of emptiness, sadness, and depression and of being rejected, unwanted, unloved, and worthless.

These findings underscore the negative implications of loneliness for mental health. Young (1982) suggests that the significant overlap between loneliness and depression mandates an adequate knowledge and understanding of loneliness if we are to deal effectively with depressed clients. Since the elderly represent an age group particularly vulnerable to loneliness due to their loss of friends and relatives, loss of major social roles (retirement, loss of spouse, etc.), and physical losses (health, mobility, etc.) resulting in emotional and social isolation, it is very important that attempts be made to assess the extent and nature of loneliness in elderly individuals.

Measurement

Recently, valid, reliable measurement of loneliness has become a major concern. Most early studies of loneliness simply asked subjects whether or not they were lonely or how often they felt lonely. This kind of global, unidimensional approach has been used extensively (Bradburn, 1969; Huyck & Hoyer, 1982; Kivett, 1979; Lowenthal, Thurner, & Chiriboga, 1975; Maisel, 1969; Shanas et al., 1968). The reliability of such self-rating measures has not been reported; but such measures obviously have content or face validity.

In recent years, several more complex, multidimensional measures of loneliness have been developed. In addition, several unidimensional measures have been developed but have not been published. These include Eddy's (1961) 24-item global measure of intensity of loneliness, which relies on a Q-sort response format and Sisenwein's (1964) 75-item measure, which built upon Eddy's earlier instrument but abandoned the Q-sort response format in favor of a four-point scale of how often respondents feel the way described in each state (i.e., often, sometimes, rarely, or never). Such measures appear to be fairly reliable; however, discriminant validity is a serious issue, considering high correlations of scores on such measures and measures of self-esteem, anxiety, and depression.

Three unidimensional measures of loneliness have been published and shown to be reliable:

1. The Abbreviated Loneliness Scale (ABLS) (see Appendix 3-C) developed by Paloutzian and Ellison (1979) consists of seven items, three of which are worded in a negative or lonely direction and four worded in a positive or nonlonely direction. Two items ask directly whether the respondent feels lonely and, if so, how often. Respondents indicate how often they feel the way described in each statement, using a four-point scale ranging from "never" to "often." Data gathered with the ABLS from middle-aged women (N = 111) showed a high correlation with another major loneliness measure, the UCLA Scale (r = .86, p < .001). Test-retest reliability of the ABLS with 121 subjects and one week between testing was r = .85 (p < .001) with an alpha coefficient of .67 (Paloutzian & Ellison, 1982). Criterion validity is supported by high correlations between the ABLS and measures of self-esteem (r = -.57), social skills (r = -.55), and a list of emotional experiences when lonely (helpless, depressed, empty, worthless, unloved, etc.) (Paloutzian & Ellison, 1982). A correlation of .61 was found between scores on the scale and a single item asking respondents how lonely they felt (Russell, 1982).

2. The Young Loneliness Inventory (see Appendix 3-C) developed by Young (1979a) is an 18-item multiple-choice self-report instrument with a format very similar to the Beck Depression Inventory. Designed as a measure of long-term loneliness, The Young Loneliness Inventory consists of items relating to social relationships, including sexual relationships; it assesses the perceived presence or absence of such relationships, as well as one's success or failure in them. Directions ask respondents to choose the one statement from a group of four that best describes themselves. Each item is scored 0 to 3, resulting in a total score ranging from a high of 0 to a low of 54. The following is a sample item:

   0. I am confident about the way I relate to men and women.

   1. I sometimes question whether there is something wrong with the way I relate to men and women.

   2. I often criticize myself for faults that seem to turn men or women off.

   3. I'm extremely disturbed that I am so undesirable to other people.

Young (1979b) reported high reliability of his measure, based on a sample of college students and a clinic sample (alpha coefficients from .78 to .84); and Primakoff (1980) reported a coefficient alpha of .79 based on use of the Young Loneliness Inventory with single adults. "Known group" validity of the inventory has been established by substantially higher loneliness scores on the measure for outpatients in a mood clinic as compared to "normals."

3. The New York University (NYU) Loneliness Scale, developed by Rubenstein and Shaver (1979), is composed of eight items that explicitly ask how lonely a person feels and how often. (See Appendix 3-C.) Items are scored on a four-point, five-point, six-point, or seven-point scale. A total loneliness score is computed by transforming each item into a standard score or z score and adding the z scores together; the scores range from   low scores below 0 to high scores above 0, with a score of 0 being average. When compared with responses from a questionnaire survey in newspapers in New York City and Worcester, Massachusetts, Rubenstein and Shaver reported coefficient alphas of .88 and .89 for their scale (Russell, 1982), thereby demonstrating the reliability of their instrument. To determine criterion validity, they compared scores on their loneliness measure with scores on measures of self-esteem and reported a correlation of $r = .59$ (Russell, 1982).

The two most often used nonpublished multidimensional measures of loneliness are Bradley's (1969) Loneliness Scale, which consists of 38 statements describing loneliness and belonging; and Belcher's (1973) Extended Loneliness Scale, which consists of 60 items and eight overlapping factors: Alienation, Anomie, Estrangement, Existential Loneliness, Loneliness Anxiety, Depression, Pathological Loneliness, and Separateness.

One of the few published multidimensional loneliness scales was devised by deJong-Gierveld and her associates (deJong-Gierveld, 1978). (See Appendix 3-C.) According to deJong-Gierveld and Raadschelders (1982), "loneliness concerns the manner in which the person perceives, experiences, and evaluates his or her isolation and lack of communication with other people" (pp. 108–109). Based on their conceptual and theoretical notions regarding the complex nature of loneliness, as well as on content analyses of life histories of 114 lonely men and women, deJong-Gierveld and her associates devised 38 items, scored on a six-point Likert scale, to measure four components of loneliness: Emotional Characteristics—items that refer to the absence of positive emotions, such as happiness and affection, and the presence of negative ones, such as fear and uncertainty; Types of Deprivation—items regarding the types of relationships that are missing and feelings associated with the deprivation of essential relationships, such as emptiness and abandonment; Time Perspective—items tapping the extent to which loneliness is experienced as unchangeable or temporary; and Personal Capabilities to Resolve Loneliness—items that assess the extent to which the cause of loneliness or its resolution is attributed to self or others (deJong-Gierveld & Raadschelders, 1982). Scale items include, "I miss having people around me" (Deprivation) and, "Times of loneliness always go away" (Time Perspective).

As reported by Russell (1982), a factor analysis of responses to the deJong-Gierveld scale by a sample of men and women from the Netherlands confirmed its multidimensional nature. The factors corresponding to each of the four components were generally reliable, with coefficient alphas ranging from .64 to .87. deJong-Gierveld and her associates also found their scale to have criterion and concurrent validity. An overall loneliness score, obtained by summing responses to all questions, correlated .49 with self-rated loneliness (obtained from a unidimensional self-report measure) and .40 with "other-rated loneliness" (obtained from a rating by a close friend) (Russell, 1982).

Probably the best known, most widely accepted, and most frequently used measure of loneliness is the UCLA Loneliness Scale developed by Russell and his colleagues (Russell et al., 1980; Russell, Peplau, & Ferguson, 1978). In developing their measure, Russell and his colleagues sought to create an instrument that would capture "the common themes that characterize the experience of loneliness for a broad spectrum of individuals"; their aim was to devise a "psychometrically adequate, easily administered, and generally available scale" (1982, p. 90). In constructing the scale, they originally chose 25 items from Sisenwein's (1964) 75-item scale and administered them to a group of 12 volunteers recruited to participate in a discussion group on loneliness for three weeks (the clinical sample) and a student sample of 192 recruited from psychology courses. The individuals responded to each item on a 5-point Likert scale. They also described their current affective state by making intensity ratings of feelings of restlessness and of feeling empty, depressed, and bored (Russell, 1982).

The final UCLA Loneliness Scale consists of the 20 items that had the highest item-total correlations (all above .50). Each item asks respondents to indicate how often they feel a particular way. Responses include often, sometimes, rarely, and never. All items are worded negatively, and often responses are coded 4, so that the total score arrived at by summing responses ranges from a low of 0 (no loneliness) to a high of 20 (great loneliness).

Sample items include, "I have nobody to talk to," and, "I cannot tolerate being so alone."

The UCLA Loneliness Scale has high internal consistency with a coefficient alpha of .96 (Russell, 1982) and a coefficient of .90 for a sample of students from Wake Forest (Solano, 1980). Based on a study of 102 University of Tulsa students conducted by Jones (1982), the scale has a test-retest reliability of .73 over a two-month period, which suggests stability of the measure over time. Recent data gathered at UCLA (Cutrona, 1982) has indicated a test-retest reliability of .62 over a seven-month period.

Several studies have demonstrated the validity of the UCLA Loneliness Scale. Solano (1980) reported a correlation of .74 between the scale and a multidimensional measure of loneliness, the Bradley Loneliness Scale. Ellison and Paloutzian (1979) similarly found a high correlation (.72) between their Abbreviated Loneliness Scale and the UCLA Scale. Jones, Freeman, and Goswick (1981) recently provided additional support for the validity of the UCLA scale when they demonstrated correlations between its scores and various personality characteristics. Lonely people, as measured by the score on the UCLA Loneliness Scale, exhibited greater self-consciousness, higher anxiety, greater social isolation, and greater shyness, and they felt less accepted by others, compared with the nonlonely. Russell et al. (1978) reported a high correlation between the UCLA scale score and a subjective self-report question about current loneliness (r (45) = .79, p < .001). They also found that those who volunteered for a loneliness clinic scored considerably higher (mean score = 0.60) than those in the comparison sample (mean score = 39.01), thus providing further evidence of the validity of the measure. The UCLA scale has also been shown to correlate highly with the Beck Depression Scale (Beck, 1967) and with the anxiety subscale of the Multiple Affect Adjective Checklist (Zuckerman & Lubin, 1965). Final support for the validity of the UCLA scale comes from Russell and his colleagues (1978) who reported significant high correlations between high scores on their measure and such feelings as boredom, emptiness, shyness, and awkwardness and low correlations with happiness. Unlike most other scales developed to measure loneliness, the UCLA Loneliness Scale has also been validated with older individuals (Perlman et al., 1978; Schultz & Moore, 1982).

Even though the UCLA Scale has been found to be reliable and valid, Russell and his colleagues have revised the scale to correct for a possible systematic response bias, due to the fact that all items on the original scale were negatively worded, and also to obtain greater discriminant validity (the original scale was highly correlated with the Beck Depression Inventory). The Revised UCLA Loneliness Scale (see Appendix 3-C) consists of 20 items, 10 negatively worded items from the original scale and 10 new positively worded items derived from a set of 19 given to 192 UCLA students (the latter 10 correlated highest with a self-report measure of loneliness administered to the same sample). The scoring is identical to that of the original scale. The revised scale has demonstrated high internal consistency, with a coefficient alpha of .94 (Russell et al., 1980). Concurrent validity of the revised scale was demonstrated by Russell, Peplau, and Cutrona (1980) who found a correlation of .62 with scores on the Beck Depression Inventory and r's above .40 with feelings of being abandoned, self-enclosed, and unsatisfied. Discriminant validity has also been demonstrated for the measure (Russell, 1982).

STRESS

Accurate assessment of the level of stress and of the impact of stress on the elderly individual is important in the overall assessment of the elderly's personal well-being and vulnerability to suicide. Based on the assumption that change is stressful because it causes divergence from a homeostatic state and necessitates adaptation, Holmes and Rahe (1967), two researchers from the University of Washington at Seattle, developed their well-known stress scale called the Schedule of Recent Events (SRE). (See Appendix 3-D.) The SRE is a 43-item checklist of common changes and life events that is quickly administered and easily understood. The instrument uses psychometrically derived, standardized weights to assess degree of change for life events that function as precursors of major illness. In developing the instrument, Holmes and Rahe placed an arbitrary value of 50 points worth of stress on the change caused by getting married. They then had thousands of individuals from a variety of different ages, backgrounds, and social classes rank the stress of the other 42 items in relation to the 50-point rating assigned to marriage. The result was a 43-item checklist that weighted death of a spouse as most stressful (100 points), Christmas and vacations least stressful (12 and 13 points, respectively), and all other events somewhere in between.

To obtain a person's "stress temperature," the person checks off those events that have occurred in the past two years, as well as those that occurred earlier if they are still thought about "a lot," to obtain a total score. The total score, or "life crisis unit" as Holmes and Rahe call it, can range from 0 to over 300 points. A score under 150 indicates low stress; 150 to 300 indicates moderate stress; and over 300 indicates high stress.

Holmes and Rahe claim that the SRE measures susceptibility to physical disease. Disruptive life events alter the steady state of psychosocial adjustment. The larger the number of such events, the greater the susceptibility to illness. In fact, research on heart patients and navy personnel conducted by Rubin and Rahe (1974) has convincingly demonstrated that changes in life events produce changes in neuroendocrine activity. Since 1967, literally hundreds of studies have substantiated the link between stress and physical and mental illness, using the SRE (Poon, 1980).

The life events approach to stress measurement, tapping a broad range of stress experiences, measures "presumptive" stress. More recent approaches to stress measurement attempt to assess "subjective" stress by ascertaining the individual's perception of each event as either positive or negative and by obtaining a self-report of the importance (impact) of each event. These approaches, which are essentially attempts to extend and refine the SRE, serve to further define the parameters of stress.

The Life Events Questionnaire (LEQ), developed by Horowitz and Wilner (1980) at the Center for the Study of Neuroses at the Langley Porter Institute, expands the 43-item SRE to 138 items and, in addition, requires subjects to assess recency and impact of each event. (See Appendix 3-D.) The LEQ also contains items on sexuality and change in sexual attachment, items not included in the Holmes and Rahe instrument. The LEQ is comprised of 11 different dimensions (marital/dating, family, finances, legal, work, home, nonfamily relations, personal, school, health of family and friends, thoughts and feelings). Subjects check each event that has occurred and indicate one of five times at which the event has occurred (one week, one month, six months, one year, or three years earlier). Respondents then indicate for each event checked whether they felt positively or negatively about it and how much they thought about it (i.e., how intrusive each event was in their thoughts).

Using the LEQ, it is possible to compute positive and negative stress preoccupation scores, as well as an overall stress score. The LEQ uses differential weights for recency and remoteness of events, as well as for each event itself. Thus, recent death of a spouse is scored higher than death of a spouse three years ago. Scoring involves summing the points for all events, taking into account the recency of each, to derive a total stress score. Reliability estimates for the LEQ are reasonably high (Horowitz & Wilner, 1980).

Horowitz and Wilner (1980) have also developed a measure of subjective distress called the Impact of Event Scale (IES). (See Appendix 3-D.) Items for the scale were derived from statements most frequently made by patients who visited their clinic after recently experiencing a seriously disturbing life event. Based on clinical work, the scale focuses on the quality of conscious experiences during the previous seven days, and the disturbing life event serves as a written referent for the scale itself (Horowitz & Wilner, 1980).

The IES consists of 16 items with 2 subscales: intrusion items and avoidance items. For the event experienced, the respondent indicates whether in the previous seven days the respondent felt in any of the following ways: "I had waves of strong feelings about it" (Intrusion), "I wished to banish it from my store of memories" (Avoidance), and so forth. The IES scores enable one to make a judgment of the qualitative level of distress and to separate those who are experiencing low levels of distress from those who are moderately or highly distressed. Horowitz and Wilner (1980) report test-retest reliability of .87 for the IES, using Cronbach's alpha (.78 for intrusion and .82 for avoidance subscores).

CONCLUSIONS

Measures of stress, such as the ones described above, should be used with caution, and only in conjunction with other more direct forms of clinical assessment. Recent studies indicate that many factors influence our perceptions of stress, as well as our ability to cope effectively. A thorough knowledge of the elderly client's past life, experiences, means of coping, health status, family and friendship support systems, and present financial status is essential for accurate   interpretation and utilization of the results obtained from stress tests.

A similar caveat is in order regarding use of depression scales, morale and life satisfaction indexes, and loneliness measures. The assessment of morale or life satisfaction, loneliness, and stress in the elderly is an important element in the overall assessment of the mental health status of older adults; it should therefore be done in conjunction with and in addition to assessment of depression in the aged.

Accurate assessment of mood, emotional state, and vulnerability to suicide depends on careful use of a broad range of techniques discussed in Part I. Pen-and-paper tests cannot take the place of a caring human being who asks appropriate questions and listens. However, such instruments can provide helpful aids for the concerned caregiver and develop valuable information that can be used in making an appropriate evaluation of vulnerability.

REFERENCES

Adams, D. L. (1969). Analysis of a life satisfaction index. *Journal of Gerontology, 24,* 470–474.

Beck, A. T. (1967). *Depression.* New York: Hoeber.

Belcher, M. J. (1973). *The measurement of loneliness: A validation of the Belcher extended loneliness scale (BELS).* Unpublished doctoral dissertation, Illinois Institute of Technology, Chicago, Ill.

Berg, S., Mellstrom, D., Persson, G., & Svanborg, A. (1981). Loneliness in the Swedish aged. *Journal of Gerontology, 36*(3), 342–349.

Bradburn, N. M. (1969). *The structure of psychological well-being.* Chicago: Aldine.

Bradley, R. (1969). *Measuring loneliness.* Unpublished doctoral dissertation, Washington State University, Pullman, Wash.

Bragg, M. (1979). *A comparative study of loneliness and depression.* Unpublished doctoral dissertation, University of California, Los Angeles, Calif.

Burnside, I. (1980). Symptomatic behaviors in the elderly. In J. E. Birren & R. B. Sloane (Eds.), *Handbook of mental health and aging* (pp. 719–742). Englewood Cliffs, N.J.: Prentice-Hall.

Cavan, R. S., Burgess, E. W., Havighurst, J., & Goldhammer, H. (1949). *Personal adjustment in old age.* Chicago, Ill.: Science Research Associates.

Cutrona, C. E. (1982). Transition to college: Loneliness and the process of social adjustment. In L. A. Peplau & D. Perlman (Eds.), *Loneliness: A sourcebook of current theory, research, and therapy* (pp. 291–309). New York: John Wiley & Sons.

deJong-Gierveld, J. (1978). The construct of loneliness: Components and measurement. *Essence,* 2(4), 221–237.

deJong-Gierveld, J., & Raadschelders, R. (1982). Types of loneliness. In L. A. Peplau & D. Perlman (Eds.), *Loneliness: A sourcebook of current theory, research, and therapy* (pp. 105–122). New York: John Wiley & Sons.

Derlega, V. J., & Margulis, S. T. (1982). Why loneliness occurs: The interrelationship of social-psychological and privacy concepts. In L. A. Peplau & D. Perlman (Eds.), *Loneliness: A sourcebook of current theory, research, and therapy* (pp. 152–165). New York: John Wiley & Sons.

Eddy, P. D. (1961). *Loneliness: A discrepancy within the phenomenological self.* Unpublished doctoral dissertation, Adelphi University, Garden City, N. Y.

Ellison, C. W., & Paloutzian, R. F. (1979, May). *Emotional, behavioral, and physical correlates of loneliness.* Paper presented at the UCLA research conference on loneliness, Los Angeles, Calif.

Flanders, J. P. (1976). From loneliness to intimacy. In J. P. Flanders (Ed.), *Practical Psychology* (23–43). New York: Harper & Row.

Fromm-Reichmann, F. (1959). Loneliness. *Psychiatry, 22,* 1–15.

George, L. K., & Bearon, L. B. (1980). *Quality of life in older persons: Meaning and measurement.* New York: Human Sciences Press.

Graney, M. (1975). Happiness and social participation in aging. *Journal of Gerontology, 30,* 701–706.

Havighurst, R. J. (1951). Validity of the Chicago attitude inventory as a measure of personal adjustment in old age. *Journal of Abnormal and Social Psychology, 46,* 24–29.

Havighurst, R. J. (1961). The nature and value of meaningful free-time activity. In R. Kleemier (Ed.), *Aging and leisure* (pp. 309–344). New York: Oxford University Press.

Holmes, T. H., & Rahe, R. H. (1967). The social readjustment rating scale. *Journal of Psychosomatic Research, 11,* 213–218.

Horowitz, M. J., & Wilner, N. (1980). Life events, stress, and coping. In L. Poon (Ed.), *Aging in the 1980's: Psychological issues* (pp. 363–373). Washington, D.C.: American Psychological Association.

Huyck, M. H., & Hoyer, W. J. (1982). *Adult development and aging.* Belmont, Calif.: Wadsworth.

Hyams, D. E. (1969). Psychological factors in rehabilitation of the elderly. *Gerontologica Clinica, 11,* 129–136.

Janke, W., & Baltisson, R. (1979). Critical consideration on methods of assessing emotional and motivational characteristics of old persons. In F. Hoffmeister & C. Muller (Eds.), *Brain function in old age* (pp. 214–227). Berlin, Germany: Springer-Verlag.

Jones, W. H. (1982). Loneliness and social behavior. In L. A. Peplau & D. Perlman (Eds.), *Loneliness: A sourcebook of current theory, research, and therapy* (pp. 238–254). New York: John Wiley & Sons.

Jones, W. H., Freeman, J. R., & Goswick, R. A. (1981). The persistence of loneliness: Self and other rejection. *Journal of Personality, 49*, 27–48.

Kivett, V. R. (1979). Discriminators of loneliness among the rural elderly: Implications for intervention. *Gerontologist, 19*, 108–115.

Knapp, M. R. J. (1977). The activity theory of aging: An examination in the English context. *Gerontologist, 17*(6), 553–559.

Kutner, F., Fanshel, D., Togo, A., & Langner, T. (1956). *Five hundred over sixty.* New York: Russell Sage Foundation.

Lawton, M. P. (1972). The dimensions of morale. In D. Kent, R. Kastenbaum, & S. Sherwood (Eds.), *Research planning and action for the elderly* (pp. 144–165). New York: Behavioral Publications.

Lawton, M. P. (1975). The Philadelphia geriatric morale scale. *Journal of Gerontology, 30*, 85–89.

Leiderman, P. H. (1980). Pathological loneliness: A psychodynamic interpretation. In J. Hartog, J. R. Audy, & Y. Cohen (Eds.), *The anatomy of loneliness* (pp. 377–393). New York: International Universities Press.

Lohmann, N. (1977). Correlations of life satisfaction, morale, and adjustment measures. *Journal of Gerontology, 32*, 73–75.

Loucks, S. (1980). Loneliness, affect and self-concept: Construct validity of the Bradley loneliness scale. *Journal of Personality Assessment, 44*(2), 124–147.

Lowenthal, M. F., Thurner, M., & Chiriboga, D. (1975). *Four stages of life: A comparative study of men and women facing transition.* San Francisco, Calif: Jossey-Bass.

Maisel, R. (1969). *Report of the continuing audit of public attitudes and concerns.* Boston: Harvard Medical School Laboratory of Community Psychiatry.

Mangen, D. J. (1977, November). *Non-random measurement error in the Bradburn affect-balance scale: Toward the development of a social historical theory of measurement error.* Paper presented at the 30th annual meeting of the Gerontological Society of America, San Francisco, Calif.

Moriwaki, S. Y. (1974). The affect-balance scale: A validity study with aged samples. *Journal of Gerontology, 29*(1), 73–78.

Morris, J. N., & Sherwood, S. (1975). A retesting and modification of the Philadelphia geriatric center morale scale. *Journal of Gerontology, 30*, 77–84.

Morris, J. N., Wolf, R. S., & Klerman, L. V. (1975). Common themes among morale and depression scales. *Journal of Gerontology, 30*(2), 209–215.

Moustakas, C. E. (1972). *Loneliness and love.* Englewood Cliffs, N.J.: Prentice-Hall.

National Council on the Aging. (1975). *The myth and reality of aging in America.* Washington, D.C.: Author.

Neugarten, B. L., Havighurst, R. J., & Tobin, S. S. (1961). The measurement of life satisfaction. *Journal of Gerontology, 16*, 134–143.

Oltman, A. M., Michals, T. J., & Steer, R. A. (1980). Structure of depression in older men and women. *Clinical Psychology, 36*, 672–675.

Paloutzian, R. F., & Ellison, C. W. (1979, May). *Developing an abbreviated loneliness scale.* Paper presented at the UCLA research conference on loneliness, Los Angeles, Calif.

Paloutzian, R. F., & Ellison, C. W. (1982). Loneliness, spiritual well-being, and the quality of life. In L. A. Peplau & D. Perlman (Eds.), *Loneliness: A sourcebook of current theory, research, and therapy* (pp. 224–237). New York: John Wiley & Sons.

Peplau, L. A., & Perlman, D. (Eds.). (1982). *Loneliness: A sourcebook of current theory, research, and therapy.* New York: John Wiley & Sons.

Perlman, D., Gerson, A., & Spinner, B. (1978). *Loneliness among senior citizens: An empirical report.* Paper presented at the 88th annual convention of the American Psychological Association, Toronto, Canada.

Poon, L. W. (Ed.). (1980). *Aging in the 1980's: Psychological issues.* Washington, D.C.: American Psychological Association.

Primakoff, L. (1980). *Patterns of living alone: A cognitive behavioral ethology.* Unpublished doctoral dissertation, University of Texas, Austin.

Rubenstein, C. M., & Shaver, P. (1979). Loneliness in two northeastern cities. In J. Hartog, J. R. Audy, & Y. Cohen (Eds.), *The anatomy of loneliness* (pp. 319–337). New York: International Universities Press.

Rubenstein, C. M., & Shaver, P. (1982). The experience of loneliness. In L. A. Peplau & D. Perlman (Eds.), *Loneliness: A sourcebook of current theory, research, and therapy* (pp. 206–223). New York: John Wiley & Sons.

Rubin, R. T., & Rahe, R. H. (1974). U. S. Navy underwater demolition team training: Biochemical studies. In E. K. E. Gunderson & R. H. Rahe (Eds.), *Life stress and illness* (pp. 208–226). Springfield, Ill.: Charles C Thomas.

Rubin, Z. (1979). Seeking a cure for loneliness. *Psychology Today, 13,* 82–90.

Russell, D. (1982). The measurement of loneliness. In L. A. Peplau & D. Perlman (Eds.), *Loneliness: A sourcebook of current theory, research, and therapy* (pp. 81–104). New York: John Wiley & Sons.

Russell, D., Peplau, L. A., & Cutrona, C. E. (1980). The revised UCLA loneliness scale: Concurrent and discriminant validity evidence. *Journal of Personality and Social Psychology, 39*(3), 472–480.

Russell, D., Peplau, L. A., & Ferguson, M. L. (1978). Developing a measure of loneliness. *Journal of Personality Assessment, 42*(3), 290–294.

Sadler, W., & Johnson, T. (1980). From loneliness to anomie. In J. Hartog, J. R. Audy, & Y. Cohen (Eds.), *The anatomy of loneliness* (pp. 36–64). New York: International Universities Press.

Schultz, N. R., & Moore, D. (1982, November). *Loneliness, correlates, attributions, and coping among older adults.* Paper presented at the annual meeting of the Gerontological Society of America, Boston, Mass.

Schwab, J. J., Holzer, C. E., & Warheit, G. J. (1973). Depressive symptomatology and age. *Psychosomatics, 14,* 135–141.

Sermat, V. (1978). Sources of loneliness. *Essence, 2,* 271–276.

Shanas, E., Townsend, P., Wedderburn, D., Friis, H., Milhoj, P., & Stenhouwer, J. (1968). *Old people in three industrial societies.* New York: Atherton.

Siegler, I. C., Nowlin, J. B., & Blumenthal, J. A. (1980). Health and behavior: Methodological considerations for adult development and aging. In L. Poon (Ed.), *Aging in the 1980's: Psychological issues* (pp. 599–612). Washington, D.C.: American Psychological Association.

Sisenwein, R. J. (1964). *Loneliness and the individual as viewed by himself and others.* Unpublished doctoral dissertation, Columbia University, New York.

Solano, C. H. (1980). Two measures of loneliness: A comparison. *Psychological Reports, 46,* 23–28.

Sullivan, H. S., (1953). *The interpersonal theory of psychiatry.* New York: W. W. Norton.

Weeks, D. G., Michela, J. C., Peplau, L. A., & Bragg, M. E. (1980). The relation between loneliness and depression: A structural equation analysis. *Journal of Personality and Social Psychology, 39,* 1238–1244.

Weiss, R. S. (Ed.). (1973). *Loneliness: The experience of emotional and social isolation.* Cambridge, Mass.: MIT Press.

Wenz, F. V. (1977). Seasonal suicide attempts and forms of loneliness. *Psychological Reports, 40,* 807–810.

Wilmott, C. J., & Vaddadi, K. S. (1981). Self-report measures of mood and morale in elderly depressives. *British Journal of Psychiatry, 138,* 230–235.

Wood, L. (1978). Loneliness, social identity, and social structure. *Essence, 2,* 259–276.

Young, J. E. (1982). Loneliness, depression and cognitive therapy: Theory and application. In L. A. Peplau & D. Perlman (Eds.), *Loneliness: A sourcebook of current theory, research, and therapy* (pp. 379–406). New York: John Wiley & Sons.

Young, J. E. (1979a, September). *An instrument for measuring loneliness.* Paper presented at the annual meeting of the American Psychological Association, New York.

Young, J. E. (1979b). Loneliness in college students: A cognitive approach (Doctoral dissertation, University of Pennsylvania). *Dissertation Abstracts International.*

Zemore, R., & Eames, N. (1979). Psychic and somatic symptoms of depression among young adults, institutionalized aged and noninstitutionalized aged. *Journal of Gerontology, 34,* 716–722.

Zilboorg, G. (1938). Loneliness. *Atlantic Monthly, 161,* 45–54.

Zuckerman, M., & Lubin, B. (1965). *Manual for the multiple affect adjective checklist.* San Diego, Calif.: Educational and Industrial Testing Service.

Appendix 3-A

A Scale To Assess Depression

Zung Self-Rating Depression Scale (SDS)

Name Age_____ Sex_____ Date_____	*None or a little of the time*	*Some of the time*	*Good part of the time*	*More or all of the time*
1. I feel down-hearted, blue and sad.				
2. Morning is when I feel the best.				
3. I have crying spells or feel like it.				
4. I have trouble sleeping through the night.				
5. I eat as much as I used to.				
6. I enjoy looking at, talking to, and being with attractive women/men.				
7. I notice that I am losing weight.				
8. I have trouble with constipation.				
9. My heart beats faster than usual.				
10. I get tired for no reason.				
11. My mind is as clear as it used to be.				
12. I find it easy to do the things I used to.				
13. I am restless and can't keep still.				
14. I feel hopeful about the future.				
15. I am more irritable than usual.				
16. I find it easy to make decisions.				
17. I feel that I am useful and needed.				

Name_____ Age_____ Sex_____ Date_____	*None or a little of the time*	*Some of the time*	*Good part of the time*	*More or all of the time*
18. My life is pretty full.	_____	_____	_____	_____
19. I feel that others would be better off if I were dead.	_____	_____	_____	_____
20. I still enjoy the things I used to do.	_____	_____	_____	_____

SDS raw score:_____

SDS index:_____

Appendix 3-B

Scales To Assess
Morale and Life Satisfaction

Philadelphia Geriatric Center Morale Scale

Key: Score 1 point for each correct response.

		Correct Response	Lawton Revision	Items Used in Morris and Sherwood Revision
1.	Things keep getting worse as I get older.	No	*	*
2.	I have as much pep as I did last year.	Yes	*	*
3.	How much do you feel lonely (not much, a lot)?	Not much	*	
4.	Little things bother me more this year.	No	*	*
5.	I see enough of my friends and relatives.	Yes	*	*
6.	As you get older you are less useful.	No	*	*
7.	If you could live where you wanted to, where would you live?	Here		
8.	I sometimes worry so much that I can't sleep.	No	*	*
9.	As I get older, things are (better, worse, same) than I thought they would be.	Better	*	*
10.	I sometimes feel that life isn't worth living.	No	*	*
11.	I am as happy now as I was when I was younger.	Yes	*	*
12.	Most days I have plenty to do.	No		
13.	I have a lot to be sad about.	No	*	*
14.	People had it better in the old days.	No		
15.	I am afraid of a lot of things.	No	*	*
16.	My health is (good, not so good).	Good	*	*

From "The Dimensions of Morale" by M. P. Lawton, in *Research Planning for the Elderly*, ed. D. Kent, R. Kastenbaum, and S. Sherwood, 1972, New York: Behavioral Publications. Copyright 1972 by Human Sciences Press. Reprinted with permission. And "A Retesting and Modification of the Philadelphia Geriatric Center Morale Scale" by J.N. Morris and S. A. Sherwood, 1975, *Journal of Gerontology, 15*. Copyright 1975 by Human Sciences Press. Reprinted with permission.

| | | Correct Response | Items Used in | |
			Lawton Revision	Morris and Sherwood Revision
17.	I get mad more than I used to.	No	*	*
18.	Life is hard for me most of the time.	No	*	*
19.	How satisfied are you with your life today (not satisfied, satisfied)?	Satisfied	*	*
20.	I take things hard.	No	*	*
21.	A person has to live for today and not worry about tomorrow.	Yes		
22.	I get upset easily.	No	*	*

Cavan Attitude Inventory

Item	*Correct Response[a]*

Health subscale

1. I feel just miserable most of the time.	Disagree
2. I am perfectly satisfied with my health.	Agree
3. I never felt better in my life.	Agree
4. If I can't feel better soon, I would just as soon die.	Disagree
5. When I was younger, I felt a little better than I do now.	Neutral[b]
6. My health is just beginning to be a burden to me.	Disagree
7. I still feel young and full of spirit.	Agree

Friendship subscale

8. I have more friends now than I ever had before.	Agree
9. I never dreamed that I could be as lonely as I am now.	Disagree
10. I would be happier if I could see my friends more often.	Neutral[b]
11. I have no one to talk to about personal things.	Disagree
12. I have so few friends that I am lonely much of the time.	Disagree
13. My many friends make my life happy and cheerful.	Agree
14. I have all the good friends anyone could wish.	Agree

Work subscale

15. I am happy only when I have definite work to do.	Agree
16. I can no longer do any kind of useful work.	Disagree
17. I am satisfied with the work I do now.	Agree
18. I have no work to look forward to.	Disagree
19. I get badly flustered when I have to hurry with my work.	Neutral[b]
20. I do better work now than ever before.	Agree
21. I have more free time than I know how to use.	Disagree

Financial subscale

22. I am just able to make ends meet.	Disagree
23. I have enough money to get along.	Agree
24. I haven't a cent in the world.	Disagree
25. All my needs are cared for.	Agree
26. I am provided with many home comforts.	Neutral[b]
27. I have everything that money can buy.	Agree
28. I have to watch how I spend every penny.	Disagree

[a] Response options for all items are Agree, Disagree, Uncertain (?).
[b] Neutral items may be answered with either agreement or disagreement and are not included in scoring the instrument.

From *Personal Adjustment in Old Age* (pp. 158–159) by R S. Cavan, E. W. Burgess, R. J. Havighurst, and H. Goldhammer, 1949, Chicago: Science Research Associates.

	Item	Correct Response[a]

Religion subscale

29.	Religion is fairly important in my life.	Agree
30.	I have no use for religion.	Disagree
31.	Religion is a great comfort to me.	Agree
32.	Religion doesn't mean much to me.	Disagree
33.	I don't rely on prayer to help me.	Disagree
34.	Religion is the most important thing in my life.	Agree
35.	Religion is only one of many interests.	Neutral[b]

Usefulness subscale

36.	I am some use to those around me.	Neutral[b]
37.	My life is meaningless now.	Disagree
38.	The days are too short for all I want to do.	Agree
39.	Sometimes I feel there's just no point in living.	Disagree
40.	My life is still busy and useful.	Agree
41.	This is the most useful period of my life.	Agree
42.	I can't help feeling now that my life is not very useful.	Disagree

Happiness subscale

43.	This is the dreariest time in my life.	Disagree
44.	I am just as happy as when I was younger.	Agree
45.	My life could be happier than it is now.	Neutral[b]
46.	I seem to have less and less reason to live.	Disagree
47.	These are the best years of my life.	Agree
48.	My life is full of worry.	Agree
49.	My life is so enjoyable that I almost wish it would go on forever.	Agree

Family subscale[c]

50.	My family likes to have me around.	Neutral[b]
51.	I am perfectly satisfied with the way my family treats me.	Agree
52.	I wish my family would pay more attention to me.	Disagree
53.	I think my family is the finest in the world.	Agree
54.	My family is always trying to boss me.	Disagree
55.	I get more love and affection now than I ever did before.	Agree
56.	My family does not really care for me.	Disagree

[c] If the respondent has no living family, the family subscale should be omitted.

Hamilton Depression Scale

Checklist of Symptoms of Depressive States

Item No.	Range of Scales	Symptom

1 0-4 Depressed mood
Gloomy attitude, pessimism about the future
Feeling of sadness
Tendency to weep
Sadness, etc 1
Occasional weeping...2
Frequent weeping...3
Extreme symptoms 4

2 0-4 Guilt
Self-reproach, feels he has let people down
Ideas of guilt
Present illness is a punishment
Delusions of guilt
Hallucinations of guilt

3 0-4 Suicide
Feels life is not worth living
Wishes he were dead
Suicidal ideas
Attempts at suicide

4 0-2 Insomnia, initial
Difficulty in falling asleep

5 0-2 Insomnia, middle
Patient restless and disturbed during the night
Waking during the night

6 0-2 Insomnia, delayed
Waking in early hours of the morning and unable to fall asleep
again

7 0-4 Work and interests
Feelings of incapacity
Listlessness, indecision and vacillation
Loss of interest in hobbies
Decreased social activities
Productivity decreased
Unable to work
Stopped working because of present illness only 4
(Absence from work after treatment or recovery may rate a
lower score.)

8 0-4 Retardation
Slowness of thought, speech, and activity
Apathy
Stupor
Slight retardation at interview 1
Obvious retardation at interview 2

Checklist of Symptoms of Depressive States

Item No.	Range of Scales	Symptom
		Interview difficult..3
		Complete stupor 4
9	0-2	Agitation Restlessness associated with anxiety
10	0-4	Anxiety psychic Tension and irritability Worrying about minor matters Apprehensive attitude Fears
11	0	Anxiety, somatic Gastrointestinal, wind, indigestion Cardiovascular, palpitations, headaches Respiratory, genitourinary, etc.
12	0-2	Somatic symptoms, gastrointestinal Loss of appetite Heavy feelings in abdomen Constipation
13	0-2	Somatic symptoms, general Heaviness in limbs, back, or head Diffuse backache Loss of energy and fatigability
14	0-2	Genital Symptoms Loss of libido Menstrual disturbances
15	0-4	Hypochondriasis Self-absorption (bodily) Preoccupation with health Querulous attitude Hypochondriacal delusions
16	0-2	Loss of weight
17	2-0	Insight
		Loss of insight..2
		Partial or doubtful loss 1
		No loss..0
		(Insight must be interpreted in terms of patient's understanding and background.)
18	0-2	Diurnal variation Symptoms worse in morning or evening (note which it is).
19	0-4	Depersonalization and derealization Feelings of unreality ⎤ Nihilistic ideas ⎦ Specify
20	0-4	Paranoid symptoms Suspicious ⎤ Ideas of reference ⎥ Not with a Delusions of reference and persecution ⎥ depressive quality Hallucinations, persecutory ⎦ Obsessional symptoms Obsessive thoughts and compulsions, against which the patient struggles.

Kutner Morale Scale

Item	*Indicated Response Scored + 1*
1. How often do you feel there's just no point in living?	Hardly ever.
2. Things just keep getting worse and worse for me as as I get older.	Disagree.
3. How much do you regret the chances you missed during your life to do a better job of living.	Not at all.
4. All in all how much unhappiness would you say you find in life today?	Almost none.
5. On the whole, how satisfied would you say you are?	Very satisfied.
6. How much do you plan ahead the things you will be doing next week or the week after? Would you say you make many plans, a few plans, or almost none?	Many plans.
7. As you get older, would you say things seem to be worse than you thought they would be?	Better.

From *Five Hundred over Sixty* (p. 49) by B. Kutner, D. Fanshel, A. Togo, and J. Langner. © 1956 by Russell Sage Foundation. Reprinted by permission of Basic Books, Inc., Publishers.

Lohmann Life Satisfaction Scale

Item	Agree	Disagree
I feel just miserable most of the time.[a]		X
I never dreamed that I could be as lonely as I am now.[a]		X
I never felt better in my life.	X	
I have no one to talk to about personal things.[a]		X
I have so few friends that I am lonely much of the time.[a]		X
I can no longer do any kind of useful work.[a]		X
This is the most useful period of my life.[a]	X	
I have more free time than I know how to use.[a]		X
I do better work than ever before.	X	
I haven't a cent in the world.		X
I have no use for religion.		X
My life is meaningless now.[a]		X
I am just as happy as when I was younger.	X	
Sometimes I feel there is no point in living.[a]		X
I can't help feeling now that my life is not very useful.[a]		X
My life is full of worry.[a]		X
This is the dreariest time of my life.[a]		X
My life is still busy and useful.	X	
I like being the age I am.	X	
I seem to have less and less reason to live.[a]		X
Most of the things I do are boring or monotonous.[a]		X
I often feel lonely.		X
Compared to other people, I get down in the dumps too often.[a]		X
Things keep getting worse as I get older.		X
These are the best years of my life.[a]	X	
I have a lot to be sad about.[a]		X
I sometimes worry so much that I can't sleep.		X
I am as happy now as I ever was.	X	
I feel old and somewhat tired.		X
The older I get, the worse everything is.		X
My life could be happier than it is now.		X
Life is hard for me most of the time.[a]		X

[a]Item included in the 18-item form of the scale.

Affect-Balance Scale

During the past few weeks did you ever feel . . .

Positive feelings:

1. Pleased about having accomplished something?[a]
2. That things were your way?
3. Proud because someone complimented you on something you had done?
4. Particularly excited or interested in something?
5. On top of the world?

Negative feelings:

1. So restless that you couldn't sit long in a seat?
2. Bored?
3. Depressed or very unhappy?
4. Very lonely or remote from other people?
5. Upset because someone criticized you?

[a]Response options for all 10 items are yes or no.

From *The Structure of Psychological Well-Being* (p. 56) by N.M. Bradburn, 1969, Chicago: Aldine Publishing Company, Inc.

Life Satisfaction Index A

Here are some statements about life in general that people feel differently about. Would you read each statement on the list, and if you agree with it, put a check mark in the space under "agree." If you do not agree with a statement, put a check mark in the space under "disagree." If you are not sure one way or the other, put a check mark in the space under "?" Please be sure to answer every question on the list.

(Key: score one point for each response marked X)

		Agree	Disagree	?
1.	As I grow older, things seem better than I thought they would be.	X		
2.	I have gotten more of the breaks in life than most of the people I know.	X		
3.	This is the dreariest time of my life.		X	
4.	I am just as happy as when I was younger.	X		
5.	My life could be happier than it is now.		X	
6.	These are the best years of my life.	X		
7.	Most of the things I do are boring or monotonous.		X	
8.	I expect some interesting and pleasant things to happen to me in the future.	X		
9.	The things I do are as interesting to me as they ever were.	X		
10.	I feel old and somewhat tired.		X	
11.	I feel my age, but it does not bother me.	X		
12.	As I look back on my life, I am fairly well satisfied.	X		
13.	I would not change my past life even if I could.	X		
14.	Compared to other people my age, I've made a lot of foolish decisions in my life.		X	
15.	Compared to other people my age, I make a good appearance.	X		
16.	I have made plans for things I'll be doing a month or a year from now.	X		
17.	When I think back over my life, I didn't get most of the important things I wanted.		X	
18.	Compared to other people, I get down in the dumps too often.		X	
19.	I've gotten pretty much what I expected out of life.	X		
20.	In spite of what people say, the lot of the average man is getting worse, not better.		X	

From *Aging in America: Readings in Social Gerontology* (pp. 141–142) by C. S. Kart and B. B. Manard, 1976, New York: Alfred Publishing. Reprinted by permission of *The Gerontologist, 16* (11), Spring 1971.

Life Satisfaction Index B

Would you please comment freely in answer to the following questions?

1 What are the best things about being the age you are now?

    1 . . . a positive answer
    0 . . . . nothing good about it

2. What do you think you will be doing five years from now? How do you expect things will be different in your life from the way they are now?

    2 . . . . better, or no change
    1 . . . . contingent: "It depends."
    0 . . . . worse

3. What is the most important thing in your life right now?

    2 . . . . anything outside of self, or a pleasant interpretation of future
    1 . . . . "hanging on," keeping health or job
    0 . . . . getting out of present difficulty, or "nothing now," or reference to the past

4. How would you say you are right now, compared with the earlier periods in your life?

    2 . . . . this is the happiest time, all have been happy, or hard to make a choice
    1 . . . . some decrease in recent years
    0 . . . . earlier periods were better; this is a bad time

5. Do you ever worry about your ability to do what people expect of you, to meet demands that people make of you?

    2 . . . . . no
    1 . . . . qualified yes or no
    0 . . . . yes

6. If you could do anything you pleased, in what part of _____ would you most like to live?

    2 . . . . present location
    0 . . . . any other location

7. How often do you find yourself feeling lonely?

    2 . . . . never, hardly ever
    1 . . . . sometimes
    0 . . . . fairly often, very often

Reprinted by permission of *The Gerontologist*/the *Journal of Gerontology, 16*, pp. 141–142, "The Measurement of Life Satisfaction" by B. L. Neugarten, R. J. Havighurst, & S. S. Tobin, copyright 1961.

8. How often do you feel there is no point in living?

    2 . . . . never, hardly ever
    1 . . . . sometimes
    0 . . . . fairly often, very often

9. Do you wish you could see more of your close friends than you do, or would you like more time to yourself?

    2 . . . . o.k. as is
    1 . . . . wish could see more of friends
    0 . . . . wish more time to self

10. How much unhappiness would you say you find in your life today?

    2 . . . . almost none
    1 . . . . some
    0 . . . . a great deal

11. As you get older, would you say things seem to be better or worse than you thought they would be?

    2 . . . . better
    1 . . . . about as expected
    0 . . . . worse

12. How satisfied would you say you are with your way of life?

    2 . . . . very satisfied
    1 . . . . fairly satisfied
    0 . . . . not very satisfied

Cornell Personal Adjustment Scale

Satisfaction with life

1. All in all, how much happiness would you say you find in life today? (check one)

    _____ Almost none. (–)
    _____ Some, but not very much. (–)
    _____ A good deal. (+)

2. In general, how would you say you feel most of the time, in good spirits or in low spirits? (check one)

    _____ I am usually in good spirits. (+)
    I am in good spirits some of the time and in low spirits some of the time.
    _____ (–)
    _____ I am usually in low spirits.

3. On the whole, how satisfied would you say you are with your way of life today? (check one)

    _____ Very satisfied. (+)
    _____ Fairly satisfied. (–)
    _____ Not very satisfied. (–)
    _____ Not very satisfied at all. (–)

Dejection

4. How often do you get the feeling that your life today is not very useful? (check one)

    _____ Often. (–)
    _____ Sometimes. (–)
    _____ Hardly ever. (+)

5. How often do you find yourself "blue"? (check one)

    _____ Often. (–)
    _____ Sometimes. (–)
    _____ Hardly ever. (+)

6. How often do you get upset by the things that happen in your day-to-day living? (check one)

    _____ Often. (–)
    _____ Sometimes. (–)
    _____ Hardly ever. (+)

Reprinted by permission of *The Gerontologist*/the *Journal of Gerontology, 15,* 1960, p. 166, "The Effect of Retirement on Personal Adjustment: A Panel Analysis" by W. E. Thompson, R. F. Streib, and J. Kosa.

Hopelessness

7. These days I find myself giving up hope of trying to improve myself. (check one)

   _____ Yes. (–)
   _____ No. (+)
   _____ Undecided. (–)

8. Almost everything these days is a racket. (check one)

   _____ Yes. (–)
   _____ No. (+)
   _____ Undecided. (–)

9. How much do you plan ahead the things that you will be doing next week or the week after? (check only one)

   _____ I make many plans. (+)
   _____ I make few plans. (–)
   _____ I make almost no plans. (–)

Note: Plus and minus signs are not included in the questionnaire as it is being completed; they indicate the positive or negative nature of the item for scoring purposes.

Appendix 3-C

Scales To Assess Loneliness

Abbreviated Loneliness Scale

Please circle the choice that best indicates how often each of the following statements describes you in general:

O = Often   S = Sometimes   R = Rarely   N = Never

1. I feel like the people most important to me understand me.   O S R N

2. I feel lonely.   O S R N

3. I feel like I am wanted by the people/groups I value belonging to.   O S R N

4. I feel emotionally distant from people in general.   O S R N

5. I have as many close relationships as I want.   O S R N

6. I have felt lonely during my life.   O S R N

7. I feel emotionally satisfied in my relationship with people.   O S R N

From "Loneliness, Spiritual Well-Being, and the Quality of Life" by R. F. Paloutzian and Craig W. Ellison, in *Loneliness: A Sourcebook of Current Theory, Research, and Therapy* (p. 228), ed. L. A. Peplau and D. Perlman, 1982, New York: John Wiley & Sons. Copyright 1982 by John Wiley & Sons. Reprinted by permission of John Wiley & Sons, Inc.

Young Loneliness Inventory

On this questionnaire are groups of statements. Please read each group of statements carefully. Then pick out the one statement in each group that best describes you. Circle the number beside the statement you picked. If several statements in the group seem to apply equally well, circle each one. Be sure to read all the statements in each group before making your choice.

1. 0 When I want to do something for enjoyment, I can usually find someone to join me.
   1 Sometimes I end up doing things alone even though I'd like to have someone join me.
   2 It often bothers me that there is no one I can go out and do things with.
   3 I'm extremely disturbed that there is no one I can go out and do things with.

2. 0 I have a close group of friends nearby that I feel part of.
   1 I'm not sure that I really belong to any close group of friends nearby.
   2 It often bothers me that I don't feel part of any close group of friends nearby.
   3 I'm extremely disturbed that I don't have a close group of friends.

3. 0 I almost always have someone to be with when I do not want to be alone.
   1 I am sometimes alone when I would prefer to be with other people.
   2 It bothers me that I am often alone when I would prefer to be with other people.
   3 I'm extremely disturbed that I am alone so often.

4. 0 I have a lot in common with other people I know.
   1 I wish my values and interests, and those of other people I know, were more similar.
   2 It often bothers me that I'm different from other people I know.
   3 I'm extremely disturbed that I'm so different from other people.

5. 0 I feel that I generally fit in with people around me.
   1 I sometimes feel that I don't fit in with the people around me.
   2 I am often bothered that I feel isolated from the people around me.
   3 I'm extremely disturbed by how isolated I feel from other people.

6. 0 There is someone nearby who really understands me.
   1 I'm not sure there's anyone nearby who really understands me.
   2 It often bothers me that no one nearby understands me.
   3 I'm extremely disturbed that no one really understands me.

7. 0 I have someone nearby who is really interested in hearing about my private feelings.
   1 I'm not sure that anyone nearby is really interested in hearing about my private feelings.

From "Loneliness, Depression, and Cognitive Therapy: Theory and Application" by J. E. Young, in *Loneliness: A Sourcebook of Current Theory, Research, and Therapy* (pp. 388–390), ed. L. A. Peplau and D. Perlman, 1982, New York: John Wiley & Sons. Copyright 1982 by John Wiley & Sons. Reprinted with permission of John Wiley & Sons, Inc.

2 It often bothers me that no one nearby is really interested in hearing about my private feelings.

3 I'm extremely disturbed that no one is really interested in hearing about my private feelings.

8. 0 I can usually talk freely to close friends about my thoughts and feelings.
   1 I have some difficulty talking to close friends about my thoughts and feelings.
   2 It often bothers me that I can't seem to communicate my thoughts and feelings to anyone.
   3 I'm extremely disturbed that my thoughts and feelings are so bottled up inside.

9. 0 I have someone nearby I can really depend on when I need help and support.
   1 I'm not sure there's anyone nearby I can really depend on when I need help.
   2 It often bothers me that there is no one nearby I can really depend on when I need help and support.
   3 I'm extremely disturbed that there is no one I can depend on when I need help and support.

10. 0 There is someone nearby who really cares about me.
    1 I'm not sure there's anyone nearby who really cares about me.
    2 It often bothers me that there is no one nearby who really cares about me.
    3 I'm extremely disturbed that no one really cares about me.

11. 0 The important people in my life have not let me down.
    1 Sometimes I feel disappointed in someone I thought I could trust.
    2 I often think about the important people in my life I trusted who have let me down.
    3 I can't trust anyone anymore.

12. 0 There is someone nearby who really needs me.
    1 I'm not sure anyone nearby really needs me.
    2 It often bothers me that there is no one nearby who really needs me.
    3 I'm extremely disturbed that no one really needs me.

13. 0 I have a partner I love who loves me.
    1 I'm not sure I have nearby a partner I love who also loves me.
    2 It often bothers me that I do not have nearby a partner I love who loves me.
    3 I'm extremely disturbed that I do not have a partner I love who loves me.

14. 0 I have a satisfying sexual relationship with someone now on a regular basis.
    1 I sometimes wish that I had a satisfying sexual relationship on a regular basis.
    2 It often bothers me that I do not have a satisfying sexual relationship with anyone.
    3 I am extremely disturbed that I do not have a satisfying sexual relationship with anyone.

15. 0 I rarely think about particular times in my life when my relationships seemed better.
    1 I sometimes wish my relationships now could be more as they were at another time in my life.
    2 I am often bothered by how unsatisfactory my relationships now are compared with another time in my life.
    3 I am extremely disturbed by how poor my relationships are now compared with another time in my life.

16. 0 I rarely wish that my relationships could be more like other people's.
     1 I sometimes wish that I could have relationships that satisfied me the way other people's relationships seem to satisfy them.
     2 I often compare the satisfaction other people seem to get from their relationships with my own lack of satisfaction.
     3 I cannot stop comparing the satisfaction other people get from their relationships with my own lack of satisfaction.

17. 0 I am confident about the way I relate to men and women.
     1 I sometimes question whether there is something wrong with the way I relate to men or women.
     2 I often criticize myself for faults that seem to turn men or women off.
     3 I'm extremely disturbed that I am so undesirable to other people.

18. 0 I am confident that I will have close, satisfying relationships in the future.
     1 I sometimes question whether I will have close, satisfying relationships in the future.
     2 I feel hopeless about ever having close, satisfying relationships.

19. 0 I haven't felt lonely during the past week (including today).
     1 I've sometimes felt lonely during the past week (including today).
     2 I've often felt lonely during the past week (including today).
     3 I could barely stand the loneliness during the past week (including today).

NYU Loneliness Scale

1. When I am completely alone, I feel lonely. (five points: almost never. . .most of the time)
2. How often do you feel lonely? (seven points: all the time. . .never)
3. When you feel lonely, how lonely do you feel? (six points: extremely lonely. . .never feel lonely)
4. Compared with people your own age, how lonely do you think you are? (five points: much lonelier. . .much less lonely)

How much do you agree with each of the following (on a 4-point, agree-disagree scale):

5. I am a lonely person.
6. I always was a lonely person.
7. I always will be a lonely person.
8. Other people think of me as a lonely person.

De Jong-Gierveld Loneliness Scale

Theoretical Subdimension	Item
1a	I miss having people around me.
1a	There's actually no one who really values your company.
1a	You have actually no one you'd want to share your joy or sorrow with.
1a	I feel alone in the world.
1a	There's nobody who really cares for me.
1a	I miss good company around me.
1a	I often feel deserted.
1a	I experience an emptiness around me.
1a	There are only a few people to whom I can relate.
1a	You can no longer expect any interest, even from closest kin.
1a	Although I have good friends, I miss not having a mate.
1a	Though I have a number of contacts, I still miss a man/woman, especially mine.
1a	I miss having a companion.
1a	I miss having a really good friend.
1b	When it comes to good relations, there always remains something to be desired.
1b	A person simply has no time to visit friends and acquaintances regularly.
1b	You learn from experience that you're ultimately better off "alone."
1b	You must complain too much about being alone, that puts people off.
1b	An ideal partner can't be found anyway.
2a	I've know times of loneliness, but these times always go away.
2a	There is ultimately no hope for someone lonely in our society.
2a	You can't resolve loneliness, not even in the long run.
2a	I've known times of deep loneliness, but sooner or later you get yourself back on your feet.

From "The Construct of Loneliness: Components and Measurement" by J. de Jong-Gierveld, 1978, *Essence, 2,* pp. 226–228. Copyright 1978 by Atkinson College Press. Reprinted with permission.

Theoretical Subdimension	Item
2a	Once lonely, always lonely.
2a	The worst of all is that this situation is so endless.
2a	Everyone is lonely every once in a while.
2a	Feelings of loneliness decrease by opening yourself up to others.
2b	There's no cure for loneliness.
2b	Only a real expert could possibly help my loneliness.
2b	Where there's a will, there's a way, also for getting over loneliness.
2b	You'll be less lonely when you actively work on it yourself.
2b	People are by nature unwilling to rescue you from your loneliness.
2b	Nobody is capable of curing his loneliness himself.
2b	Loneliness can't be cured, you've got to learn to live with it.
2b	If only I had some more energy, then I could get rid of this feeling of loneliness very soon.

Revised UCLA Loneliness Scale

Directions: Indicate how often you feel the way described in each of the following statements. Circle one number for each.

Statement	Never	Rarely	Sometimes	Often
1. I feel in tune with the people around me.[a]	1	2	3	4
2. I lack companionship.	1	2	3	4
3. There is no one I can turn to.	1	2	3	4
4. I do not feel alone.[a]	1	2	3	4
5. I feel part of a group of friends.[a]	1	2	3	4
6. I have a lot in common with the people around me.[a]	1	2	3	4
7. I am no longer close to anyone.	1	2	3	4
8. My interests and ideas are not shared by those around me.	1	2	3	4
9. I am an outgoing person.[a]	1	2	3	4
10. There are people I feel close to.[a]	1	2	3	4
11. I feel left out.	1	2	3	4
12. My social relationships are superficial.	1	2	3	4
13. No one really knows me well.	1	2	3	4
14. I feel isolated from others.	1	2	3	4
15. I can find companionship when I want to.	1	2	3	4
16. There are people who really understand me.[a]	1	2	3	4
17. I am unhappy being so withdrawn.	1	2	3	4
18. People are around me but not with me.	1	2	3	4
19. There are people I can talk to.[a]	1	2	3	4
20. There are people I can turn to.[a]	1	2	3	4

Note: The total score is the sum of all 20 items.

[a]Item should be used; i.e., 1 = 4, 2 = 3, 3 = 2, 4 = 1 before scoring.

Appendix 3-D

Scales To Assess Stress

Holmes and Rahe Scale of Recent Events

Rank	Event	Average Points	Write Number of Points That Apply to You
1.	Death of spouse	100	_____
2.	Divorce	73	_____
3.	Marital separation	65	_____
4.	Jail term	63	_____
5.	Death of close family member	63	_____
6.	Personal injury or illness	53	_____
7.	Marriage	50	_____
8.	Fired at work	47	_____
9.	Marital reconciliation	45	_____
10.	Retirement	45	_____
11.	Change in health of family member	44	_____
12.	Pregnancy	40	_____
13.	Sex difficulties	39	_____
14.	Gain of new family members	39	_____
15.	Business readjustment	39	_____
16.	Change in financial state	38	_____
17.	Death of close friend	37	_____
18.	Change to different line of work	36	_____
19.	Change in number of arguments with spouse	35	_____
20.	Mortgage over $10,000[a]	31	_____
21.	Foreclosure of mortgage or loan	30	_____
22.	Change in responsibilities at work	29	_____
23.	Son or daughter leaving home	29	_____
24.	Trouble with in-laws	29	_____
25.	Outstanding personal achievement	28	_____
26.	Spouse begins or stops work	26	_____
27.	Begin or end school	26	_____
28.	Change in living conditions	25	_____
29.	Revision of personal habits	24	_____
30.	Trouble with boss	23	_____
31.	Change in work hours or conditions	20	_____
32.	Change in residence	20	_____
33.	Change in schools	20	_____
34.	Change in recreation	19	_____
35.	Change in church activities	19	_____

[a]Given inflation, we suggest you increase this to $30,000.

Reprinted with permission from the *Journal of Psychosomatic Research, 11*, pp. 213–218, T. H. Holmes & R. H. Rahe, "The Social Readjustment Rating Scale," copyright 1967, Pergamon Press, Ltd.

36. Change in social activities	18	_____
37. Mortgage or loan less than $10,000[a]	17	_____
38. Change in sleeping habits	17	_____
39. Change in number of family get-togethers	15	_____
40. Change in eating habits	15	_____
41. Vacation	13	_____
42. Christmas	12	_____
43. Minor violations of the law	11	_____

Total Points of Those Items That Apply to You   _____

Life Events Questionnaire

The checklist below consists of events that are sometimes important experiences. Read down the list until you find events that have happened to you personally. Check the box under the column that indicates how long ago the event happened. Check each event as many times as it happened. For events that continue for a long period of time, such as pregnancy, check the beginning date and the ending date and then check the boxes in between. If you can't remember the exact dates, just be as accurate as you can.[a]

Weights

	Within 0-1 mo.	Within 1-6 mo.	Within 6-12 mo.	Within 1-2 yr.	Over 2 yr.
Death of a child or spouse (husband, wife, or mate)?	90	81	67	50	32
Death of a child or spouse (husband, wife, or mate)? (2nd)	90	81	67	50	32
The death of a parent, brother, or sister?	79	70	51	34	22
The death of a parent, brother, or sister? (2nd)	79	70	51	34	22
The death of a parent, brother, or sister? (3rd)	79	70	51	34	22
The loss of a close friend or important relationship by death?	70	53	36	22	12
The loss of a close friend or important relationship by death? (2nd)	70	53	36	22	12
Legal troubles resulting in being held in jail?	82	65	51	37	27
Financial difficulties?	60	43	26	13	7
Being fired or laid off?	68	46	27	16	8
A miscarriage or abortion (patient or spouse)?	71	53	31	18	11
Divorce, or a breakup with a lover?	76	63	45	29	16
Separation from spouse because of marital problems?	75	61	41	24	14
Court appearance for a serious violation?	70	41	23	13	5
An unwanted pregnancy (patient, wife)?	72	57	42	25	15

[a]These are instructions to subjects who just indicate occurrence and frequency of events. The numbers are the weightings later applied to these subjects' check marks. Scores for internal events and external events are added separately. Investigators interested only in external events could simply delete internal events.

	Weights				
	Within 0-1 mo.	Within 1-6 mo.	Within 6-12 mo.	Within 1-2 yr.	Over 2 yr.
Hospitalization of a family member?	69	46	26	14	8
Unemployment more than one month (if regularly employed)?	57	42	20	10	6
Because of illness/injury kept in bed for week or more, hosp. or emerg. room?	65	48	25	12	5
Extramarital affair?	62	50	37	25	17
Loss of a personally valuable object?	47	26	13	8	5
Involvement in a lawsuit (other than divorce)?	61	41	23	13	7
Failing an important examination?	62	37	19	9	5
Breaking an engagement?	65	47	27	14	7
Arguments with spouse (husband, wife)?	59	40	26	17	11
Taking on a large loan?	42	29	20	14	10
Being drafted into the military?	62	51	39	30	17
Troubles with boss or other workers?	50	23	9	4	3
Separation from a close friend?	49	36	24	16	10
Taking an important examination?	45	12	5	2	2
Separation from spouse because of job?	65	51	38	26	15
A big change in work or in school?	49	30	16	9	5
A move to another town, city, state or country?	46	32	20	10	5
Getting married or returning to spouse after separation?	60	45	34	23	18
Minor violations of the law?	31	15	7	3	2
Moved residence within the same town or city?	25	13	7	3	2
Birth or adoption of a child?	52	39	26	18	15
Being confused for over three days?	62	34	15	10	
Being angry for over three days?	52	25	10	5	
Being nervous for over three days?	48	23	10	5	
Being sad for over three days?	46	24	12	6	
Spouse unfaithful?	68	55	40	27	19
Attacked, raped or involved in violence?	72	57	42	25	18

Impact of Event Scale

Instructions: Please fill in the Information Section. Below that is a list of comments made by people after stressful life events. Please fill in the box for each item, indicating how frequently these comments were true for you *during the past seven days*. If they did not occur during that time, please fill in the not-at-all box. Please answer *each* item by filling in *one* of the boxes.

Information:

About _____ ago, I experienced _____

      (weeks)   (write in life event)

		Not At All	Rarely	Some-times	Often
1.	I thought about it when I didn't mean to.	[1]	[2]	[3]	[4]
2.	I had trouble doing other things because the event kept coming into my mind.	[1]	[2]	[3]	[4]
3.	I avoided letting myself get upset when I thought about it or was reminded of it.	[1]	[2]	[3]	[4]
4.	I tried to remove it from memory.	[1]	[2]	[3]	[4]
5.	I had trouble falling asleep or staying asleep because of pictures or thoughts about it that came into my mind.	[1]	[2]	[3]	[4]
6.	I had waves of strong feelings about it.	[1]	[2]	[3]	[4]
7.	I had dreams about it.	[1]	[2]	[3]	[4]
8.	I stayed away from reminders of it.	[1]	[2]	[3]	[4]
9.	I felt as if it hadn't happened or it wasn't real.	[1]	[2]	[3]	[4]
10.	I tried not to talk about it.	[1]	[2]	[3]	[4]
11.	Pictures about it popped into my mind.	[1]	[2]	[3]	[4]
12.	Other things kept making me think about it.	[1]	[2]	[3]	[4]
13.	I was aware that I still had a lot of feelings about it, but I didn't deal with them.	[1]	[2]	[3]	[4]
14.	I tried not to think about it.	[1]	[2]	[3]	[4]
15.	Any reminder brought back feeling about it.	[1]	[2]	[3]	[4]
16.	My feelings about it were kind of numb.	[1]	[2]	[3]	[4]

Chapter 4

Assessing Suicidal Risk in the Elderly: The Role of the Practitioner

The identification of a suicidal risk is called an "assessment." The lethality potential is the probability for a successful suicide, ranging from low to moderate to high. The physician, nurse, social worker, priest or rabbi, or other caregiver who is in direct contact with the elderly can play a crucial role in the identification of the suicidal elderly and in the assessment of the lethality potential and imminence of suicide. These "gatekeepers" are often contacted by elderly individuals just prior to their self-destructive act.

Physicians are most often the ones to whom the desperate elderly turn. Over 75 percent of the elderly who commit suicide see a physician shortly before the act (Grollman, 1971; Litman, Curphey, Shneidman, Farberow, & Tabachnick, 1963; M. Miller, 1979). Barraclough (1971) found in his study of geriatric suicides in England that 70 percent of them had seen a doctor within a month before taking their own lives. M. Miller (1976) similarly found that 76 percent of the elderly male suicides he studied had seen a physician within the month prior to their death. The important role of the physician in preventing elderly suicide thus cannot be overemphasized.

Yet physicians often fail to recognize the suicide signals that their patients are giving. They are not specifically trained in medical schools or anywhere else to recognize such signals in elderly patients. In one study, Rockwell and O'Brien (1973) found that physicians lack current knowledge about suicide, but also that they desire to learn more. It is particularly interesting to note that, of the physicians surveyed in this study, only eight (14 percent) correctly identified the over-60 age group as the most vulnerable in terms of successful suicide. Most thought that those aged 30 and under most frequently killed themselves.

Many elderly who are seriously contemplating suicide visit their doctor with various somatic complaints. Some come with no apparent physical ills. Others just feel something is wrong. By taking a little time to listen to the elderly patient, paying particular attention to the tone of voice, handshake, facial expression, dress and personal grooming, and mood state, the physician might be alerted that something is seriously wrong, and that that something is not just a medical or physical problem. Physicians should carefully study the warning signs of depression and suicide in the elderly presented in Part I and be alert for them in their elderly patients. Taking the time to discover if the client has recently experienced a crisis—such as the loss of a spouse, death of a best friend, relocation, or some other event—can also alert the physician to a particularly vulnerable time for the elderly individual.

Accurate assessment of suicidal risk in the elderly depends upon adequate knowledge of relevant demographic variables, personal background and family life history of the individual, the present crisis, past crises, typical response patterns to such crises, coping strategies, past and present life styles, past and present history of physical and mental illness, resources available (financial, personal, and social), and relationships with "significant others." Accurate assessment also depends upon carefully listening to and accurately perceiving verbal communications, as well as attitudinal and behavioral changes, in the elderly individual. Finally, accurate assessment depends upon appropriate knowledge of the suicide plan and accurate assessment of lethality potential of the elderly client.

Physicians and other caregivers working with the elderly should also have a thorough knowledge of the demographic and personal background factors and life style characteristics that predispose one to commit suicide and, specifically, of precipitating factors in suicide in the elderly. In this chapter, our focus is on the accurate recognition of clues to suicide and on the evaluation of the lethality potential of the elderly individual.

CLUES TO SUICIDE

"Prodromal clues," as they are referred to by Shneidman, Farberow, and Litman (1970), are the precursors to suicide. The concept of prodromal clues to suicide is not new. Over 300 years ago, in his famous work *Anatomy of Melancholy*, Robert Burton (1652/1979) referred to the "prognostics of melancholy, or signs of things to come." These clues exist a few days, weeks, or months before the suicide. As Shneidman et al. (1970) point out, recognition of these clues is a necessary first step to lifesaving.

In his indepth investigation of 301 completed suicides, M. Miller (1978) discovered that 60 percent of them gave verbal or behavioral clues to their self-inflicted deaths. Robins, West, and Murphy (1977) similarly found in their study that two-thirds of those who eventually killed themselves had previously communicated their interest in committing suicide. Physicians in particular, but also nurses, social workers, ministers, and other caregivers who work directly with the elderly and are in a position to observe their attitudes, feelings, and behaviors, must be perceptive and sensitive to such clues and warnings of suicidal behavior.

Clues to suicide may be classified as verbal, behavioral, situational, or syndromatic (Shneidman et al., 1970). Verbal clues may be direct or indirect. Direct verbal clues include such statements as:

- I am going to kill myself.
- I'm going to commit suicide.
- I'm going to end it all.
- I want to end it all.

Direct suicidal threats should always be taken seriously. Of those who threaten suicide, 80 percent eventually kill themselves. Suicidal ideations and fantasies should also be regarded as serious clues to suicide.

Indirect verbal clues are more subtle than direct suicidal threats, but, nevertheless, signal the intention to die. Indirect verbal clues are such statements as:

- I'm tired of life.
- What's the point of going on?
- My family would be better off without me.
- Who cares if I'm dead anyway?
- I can't go on anymore.
- I'm so tired of it all.
- I just want out.
- You would be better off without me.

Some verbal clues are in coded form and require keen interpretation to detect the self-destructive interest. The following are examples of such statements:

- Soon I won't be around.
- You shouldn't be having to take care of me any longer.
- Soon you won't have to worry about me anymore.
- Goodbye, I won't be here when you return.

Behavioral clues may also be either direct or indirect. The most direct behavioral clue is a suicide attempt. Suicide attempts are obviously serious clues to suicidal behavior. One in three attempters eventually completes suicide; the figures are even higher for the elderly, most of whom kill themselves within one or two years after an attempt. Indirect behavioral clues include:

- donating body to a medical school
- purchasing a gun
- stockpiling pills
- putting personal and business affairs in order
- making or changing a will
- taking out insurance or changing beneficiaries
- making funeral plans
- giving away money and/or possessions
- changes in behavior, especially episodes of screaming or hitting, throwing things, or failure to get along with family, friends, or peers
- suspicious behavior, for example, going out at odd times of the day or night, waving or kissing good-bye (if not characteristic)
- sudden interest or disinterest in church and religion
- scheduling of appointment with doctor for no apparent physical cause or very shortly after the last visit to the doctor
- loss of physical skills, general confusion, or loss of understanding, judgment, or memory

L. Miller (1979) has identified three major areas of behavioral deviance in the elderly: self-care (negative changes in eating, toileting, and grooming behaviors), task behaviors (inability to perform various household or social tasks), and relationship behaviors (argumentative, hostile, irritable, or difficult conduct in interactions with spouse, children, friends, or neighbors). The term *geriatric delinquent* has been coined to describe the elderly person undergoing a process of social deviance. The acting-out behaviors engaged in by some in this age group may be a clue that all is not well. When a usually quiet, reserved, polite woman of 80 starts screaming and otherwise acting out in her social interactions, it is time for relatives, friends, and physician to take note.

In some cases the situation itself may be the clue to suicide in the elderly. A recent move, death of a spouse, child, or friend, or a diagnosis of terminal illness may precipitate a suicidal crisis in the elderly. The caregiver thus should be aware of recent crises in the life of the elderly individual. Recent arguments with family members or more serious problems in relationships with significant others may signal danger.

The syndromatic clues consist of those psychological syndromes (constellations of symptoms) that are most often associated with suicide. Depression, particularly when accompanied by anxiety, is the most important clue to suicide in the aged. Tension and agitation, guilt, and dependency—particularly when dependency needs are threatened or frustrated—are other important syndromatic clues. Rigidity, impulsiveness, and isolation are also clues. Accurate assessment of such syndromes in the aged is crucial in suicide prevention.

According to Pavkov (1982), the key factors in recognizing the suicidal elderly may be expressed in the mnemonic ASK:

*A*ttention to expressed suicidal interests

*S*ymptomatological variations

*K*een observation of attitudinal and/or activity change

The caregiver who deals with elderly individuals, as well as relatives and friends, should keep eyes and ears open for suicidal clues. It is important to listen to the communications and expressions of feelings of the elderly individual and to observe all changes in attitudes, activities, and daily behaviors. The physician, nurse, social worker, minister, or other caregiver who does not listen to the expression of suicidal thoughts and feelings or who fails to notice signs of depression or signals of possible suicide may actually do serious harm.

Suicide is a taboo topic that most people, including physicians, tend to avoid. The topic often arouses anxiety in physicians. For this reason, they tend to overlook signals of suicide in individuals. It is much more comfortable to just look for a physical problem, prescribe a pill or other remedy, and send the patient off to "get well." But the elderly suicidal patient often interprets such behavior in the physician as another rejection, as a lack of concern or interest, which only confirms the patient's sense of worthlessness, despair, and futility, especially if the physician is regarded as a trusted and respected caregiver. The desperate individual may assume that, because of the potential rescuer's unresponsiveness, the feeling that no one cares is indeed accurate and proceed to commit suicide. Many elderly individuals come to their physicians with somatic complaints, hoping the physicians will see the "real" problem and the individuals' anguish and despair and help before it is "too late." The physician who takes the time really to listen to the elderly individual, who exhibits genuine concern, warmth, and caring, and who goes beneath the surface and looks for problems and clues to suicide can prevent suicide in such individuals. Other caregivers to whom the desperate elderly may turn have a similar responsibility to take the time to discover the real problem and accurately to read the warning signs of suicide.

EVALUATION OF LETHALITY POTENTIAL

In evaluating lethality potential, the practitioner dealing with the elderly should first consider demographic factors. Is the individual male or female? white or nonwhite? married or widowed? living alone or with relatives? The elderly white male who is widowed and living alone in a rooming house in the inner city with no contact with friends or relatives presents the highest risk. On the other hand, an elderly nonwhite female living in an extended family system in a rural area presents a much lower risk. Other important factors are histories of previous attempts, of previous depression, or of suicide or mental illness in the family.

After determining relevant demographic factors and making a judgment of risk based on such factors, the practitioner next needs to be aware of verbal, behavioral, situational, and syndromatic clues that signal suicide in the elderly. Obviously, the more direct and numerous the communications regarding suicidal intent and ideation, the greater the danger. Alcoholism and depression are two of the most important warning signs. The mental illnesses associated with cerebral arteriosclerosis and senile dementia, especially when depressive and hypochondriacal symptoms are present, also carry a high lethality potential. The practitioner needs to be particularly sensitive to very recent changes in the environment, such as a major move, and to present crises, such as the death of a spouse or close friend, both of which can precipitate suicide.

Relations with family members and "significant others" provide additional clues to lethality potential. Suicide is usually not an individual behavior but rather a dyadic one, involving at least two people. A recent argument or breakup of a relationship with a family member signals danger. If a family member and significant others are warm and caring and there are open lines of communication, the lethality potential is less. If, on the other hand, relatives are critical and rejecting and inhibited communication and de- creased gratification characterize the relationships, the lethality potential is greatly increased.

The most important steps in evaluation of lethality potential are ascertain- ing first the existence of a suicide plan and then determining the lethality, availability, and accessibility of the method of self-destruction specified in the plan. The suicide plan can be defined as "those suicidal ideations or conceptualizations of suicide and the ways and means of suicide that can lead to the final act of taking his/her life" (Hatton, Valente, & Rink, 1977, p. 52). There are four criteria to assess in order to determine the seriousness of a suicidal plan: (1) method (Has the individual decided upon pills, hanging, or some other method?), (2) availability (Is the method available? easily accessible? possible to gain access to?), (3) specificity (Is the method concrete and definite? Is the plan all worked out regarding time, place, and other specific details?), (4) lethality (Is shooting, the most lethal method, the one chosen?).

To determine the extent and lethality potential of the suicide plan, the practitioner must ask a series of direct, straightforward questions. Many physicians and other caregivers still believe that asking directly about suicidal thoughts, feelings, or intentions will encourage the individual to commit suicide. In reality, the opposite is true. Not asking encourages suicide. When asked, most individuals readily discuss their suicidal feelings and intentions and are glad to be able to share their thoughts with someone who cares enough to ask. They can achieve great relief by bringing their suicidal intentions out into the open and sharing their tortured "secret" (Hatton et al., 1977; Pavkov, 1982; Shneidman et al., 1970).

The questions asked may be general ones, such as, "How is your life going?" If the answers to such questions suggest possible suicidal thoughts or intentions, more specific questions should then be asked. For example:

- Are you thinking of suicide?
- Have you worried about suicide?
- Do you wish you could end it all?
- Do you feel you would be better off dead?

A friendly, matter-of-fact tone of voice should be used. Questions that are "minimizing" or "negatively prompting" should be avoided (Oliven, 1951). Such inappropriate questions include:

- Just a routine question, but are you thinking of suicide?
- You aren't thinking of anything like that, but just let me ask you . . . ?

A qualified denial of suicidal intent usually indicates a low lethality potential. A hedging reply ("Who knows?"), a flood of self-accusations ("I'm not fit to live"), or an admission of intent signals high lethality potential. If such answers are given, direct questions regarding the suicide plan are essential.

To ascertain the details of the suicide plan, the practitioner must ask what particular method, if any, has been chosen. If the method is shooting, the practitioner should ask directly if the elderly individual has a gun or can easily get one. Shooting, jumping from high places, and cutting are the most lethal methods. Taking poison or analgesic or soporific substances is a less lethal method.

If a particular method has been chosen, it is important to determine, through direct questioning, how easily available and accessible such a method is. Questions about specifics of the plan are also important. Is the day and time specified? If the individual has chosen a highly lethal method, such as shooting, and has a gun already or a way to obtain one and has fixed the time and place to commit suicide, the danger is imminent. Measures to protect the person must be taken immediately. Hospitalization, antidepressants, or close supervision by a family member—or some combination of these steps—is demanded.

Two final factors must be considered in assessing the lethality potential: resources and communication. Internal resources include personality characteristics, ego strength, coping abilities and strategies, and physical health. External resources include money, family, friends, and neighborhood resources and services available to the individual. The greater the resources available to the "at-risk" individual, the lower the lethality potential and the greater the potential for successful intervention. Communication includes the extent to which the elderly individual feels able to communicate with family members, friends, and neighbors and with physicians and other caregivers regarding the individual's feelings and suicidal intentions. How easily can the individual ask for help? To what extent does the individual feel accepted and understood by others? If no open lines of communication exist, the danger of suicide is greatest.

Recognition of suicidal clues and accurate evaluation of the lethality potential may save the life of an "at-risk" elderly individual, who can then receive appropriate help. According to Shneidman et al. (1970), anyone can be a lifesaver by developing a special attitude for suicide prevention. All that is required, they suggest, is "sharp eyes and ears, a pinch of wisdom, an ability to act appropriately, and a deep resolve" (p. 439).

REFERENCES

Barraclough, B. M. (1971). Suicide in the elderly. In D. W. Kay & A. Walk (Eds.), *Recent developments in psychogeriatrics* (pp. 89–97). London: Headley Brothers.

Burton, R. (1979). *Anatomy of melancholy.* New York: Ungar Publishing Co. (Original work published 1652)

Grollman, E. (1971). *Suicide: Prevention, intervention, and postvention.* Boston: Beacon Press.

Hatton, C. L., Valente, S. M., & Rink, A. (Eds.). (1977). *Suicide: Assessment and intervention.* New York: Appleton-Century-Crofts.

Litman, R., Curphey, T., Shneidman, E., Farberow, N., & Tabachnick, N. (1963). Investigations of equivocal suicide. *Journal of the American Medical Association, 184,* 924–929.

Miller, L. (1979). Toward a classification of aging behaviors. *Gerontologist, 19,* 283–290.

Miller, M. (1976). *Suicide among older men.* Unpublished doctoral dissertation, University of Michigan, Ann Arbor.

Miller, M. (1978). Geriatric suicide: The Arizona study. *Gerontologist, 18,* 488–495.

Miller, M. (1979). *Suicide after sixty: The final alternative.* New York: Springer.

Oliven, J. F. (1951). The suicidal risk: Its diagnosis and evaluation. *New England Journal of Medicine, 245,* 488–494.

Pavkov, J. (1982). Suicide in the elderly. *Ohio's Health, 34*(1), 21–28.

Robins, L., West, P., & Murphy, G. (1977). The high rate of suicide in older white men. *Social Psychiatry, 12,* 1–20.

Rockwell, D., & O'Brien, W. (1973). Physicians' knowledge and attitudes about suicide. *Journal of the American Medical Association, 225,* 1347–1349.

Shneidman, E. S., Farberow, N. L., & Litman, R. (1970). *The psychology of suicide.* New York: Science House.

Part II

Suicide Prevention: Intervention Techniques and Strategies

Chapter 5

The Role of the Practitioner

THE NEGLECTED GENERATION

As documented in previous chapters, the elderly are particularly at risk for suicide. Multiple loss and depression, loneliness and isolation are too often companions of the old. Yet, although they have the highest rates of clinical depression and other functional disorders at the same time that their tolerances and coping strengths are waning and thus require mental health services and interventions to remain functioning and interested in life, the elderly as a group are grossly underdiagnosed, undertreated, and underhelped by the mental health profession.

A study by the National Institute of Mental Health (NIMH), reported by the World Health Organization in 1959, listed the following incidences of new cases of all types of psychopathology per 100,000 population: under age 15, 2.3; ages 25–34, 7.3; ages 35–54, 93.0; and ages above 65, 236.1 (Butler, 1975). These figures clearly indicate that the elderly are the group that is most susceptible to mental illness. Intensive studies in specific communities have similarly documented the increased need for mental health intervention for the elderly (Abrahams & Patterson, 1978; Berg, Browning, Hill, & Wenkert, 1970; Lowenthal et al., 1967).

Equally well documented is the failure of the mental health system to meet the needs of the elderly. In 1970, it was estimated that about three million older people with significant psychiatric problems did not receive help (Butler, 1975). According to the Biometry Branch of NIMH, if such trends of mental health service continue, about 80 percent of the elderly people who need assistance will never be served (Butler, 1975). Kahn (1975) suggested that, compared with past decades, we actually serve a smaller proportion of the elderly who need mental health intervention. The neglect of this population in fact is well documented in numerous recent studies (Knight, 1978–1979; Sparacino, 1978–1979; Storandt, Siegler, & Elias, 1978). Why are the elderly, the group most in need of mental health services, neglected and ignored by the mental health profession? There are several explanations. Smith (1979) rightly notes that, in writings concerned with the psychological treatment of the aging, the elderly are portrayed as "aimless, apathetic, debilitated, disruptive, hypochondriacal, insecure . . . out of control, sluggish, seclusive, and temperamental" (p. 333). The elderly are also often portrayed as rigid and unable to change, crabby and garrulous, overly dependent and clinging.

In addition to such portrayals in the psychological literature, our culture abounds with numerous other negative stereotypes of the old. The old are sexless, senile, and nonproductive. Butler (1975) suggests that psychiatry has shown a sense of futility and "therapeutic nihilism" about age (p. 20). Kastenbaum (1964) has called mental health professionals "reluctant therapists" when it comes to treating the old (p. 139). Those in the mental health field, unfortunately, hold many of the same stereotypical negative beliefs about aging and the old as others in our culture. The elderly are seen as "poor risks" for treatment because of their age. They are also viewed as "low-status" patients, as are the poor and members of various minorities. A study by the American Psychoanalytic Association showed that, of the private patients seen by its members, 98 percent were white and 78 percent were educated at the college level or higher (Hamburg et al., 1967). Other studies have confirmed these findings (Brill & Storrow, 1960; Hollingshead & Redlich, 1958; Schaffer & Myers, 1954). Schofield (1964), in a summary of research findings, called the selection of private psychiatric patients the YAVIS syndrome—those selected were young, attractive, verbal, intelligent, and successful.

Butler and Lewis (1977) suggest that "professional ageism" encompasses a number of elements: (1) therapists' fears of their own old age, (2) therapists' conflicted feelings about their parents' aging, (3) a belief that aging means inevitable decline, (4) pessimism about the likelihood of change in the older client, and (5) a view that it is futile to invest effort in a person with limited life expectancy. A report by the Group for the Advancement of Psychiatry, Committee on Aging, lists similar reasons for the therapists' negative feelings but states in addition that working with the aged may induce feelings of helplessness in the therapist or, if the patient dies, may challenge the therapist's sense of importance. Some therapists may actually be "gerophobic," demonstrating intense fear of or hatred of the aged.

Much of the writing regarding old age and the old serves to promote negative myths and stereotypes. There is a paucity of accurate information available and a lack of systematic, controlled studies. The result is that the would-be helper is often left helpless and misinformed. Also lacking is proper training and education in graduate and medical schools.

In general, the aged have historically been considered inappropriate for psychoanalytic and other insight-oriented interventions due to the belief that they are rigid, possess insufficient energy, and have stored up a well of unconscious material that would have to be uncovered before therapy could succeed. Indeed, Freud argued that psychoanalysis was not appropriate for the old, and many therapists since have tended to agree. As a result, the elderly have been underrepresented in both psychoanalysis and individual therapy.

The insufficiency and expense of mental health services have also been cited as reasons why older adults have been underserved (Gaitz, 1974; LeBray, 1979). Mental health services *are* expensive and many older adults simply cannot afford them. Yet traditional services may not be appropriate for the elderly, given their special problems, needs, concerns, and limitations.

Finally, many elderly themselves do not believe in taking their problems or personal concerns to mental health professionals. There is a stigma attached to receiving such help; and many prefer to turn to church or family members for help with their problems. For all of these reasons, direct intervention to prevent suicide in the elderly is hampered.

WORKING WITH THE OLD: A NEW FRONTIER

Psychogeriatrics is the treatment and management of mental illness in the elderly. A geropsychiatrist or geropsychologist is a psychiatrist or psychologist who works with elderly individuals who suffer from depression or other mental or emotional problems.

Today, several kinds of professionals are working with the elderly in a variety of settings and are effectively employing several different intervention techniques. Psychotherapists, psychoanalysts, psychiatrists, doctors, nurses, social caseworkers, recreational therapists, pastoral counselors, and peer counselors are all working successfully with troubled elders. Treatment settings include nursing homes, day care centers, nutrition program sites, senior centers, retirement communities, hospitals, churches, local neighborhood programs, and the community at large. Intervention strategies range from traditional psychoanalysis to psychoanalytic group work, support groups, creative therapies (art, music, dance, and drama), drug therapy, recreational and activity therapy, and reminiscence or life review therapy to more exotic techniques such as pet therapy.

In the following pages, we focus on the special needs, concerns, and problems of the elderly and on the unique personal skills, qualities, special techniques, and strategies that are necessary to make a significant positive impact on the elderly in need of help. We also review and highlight the most important contributions of the new field of psychogeriatrics as in efforts to help the elderly individual at risk of committing suicide. Most of our recommendations apply to those who are conducting individual therapy or engaged in one-on-one situations with the troubled elderly client. Drug therapy and various other group therapies and intervention strategies are dealt with separately in the following chapters.

General Considerations

(To meet effectively the mental health needs of the suicide-prone elderly, the caregiver must be aware of the impact of multiple loss (health, beauty, youth, spouse, friends, job, money) and the relationships between physical changes, pain, stress, and emotional problems.) The caregiver must also possess a good knowledge of existing myths and stereotypes about aging and the old and have an adequate understanding of the physical, psychological, economic, social, and other changes accompanying the aging process and of their impact on the elderly individual. Knowledge as to which of the elderly are most vulnerable to commit suicide, combined with a knowledge of verbal, behavioral, situational, and syndromatic clues to possible suicide, is essential to suicide prevention. The ability to recognize and assess depression, loneliness, stress, and unhappiness in the elderly is important. The caregiver should also be aware of the various counseling and psychological services, recreation programs, support and self-help groups, and other relevant services available in the local community. Finally, the caregiver should keep abreast of the literature on particular therapeutic interventions that have proven successful with the elderly suffering from depression, loneliness, and social isolation. (Many of these interventions are discussed in detail in the following chapters.)

First, however, those who want to help the suicide-prone elderly must come to terms with their own aging and death, their own relationships with parents and grandparents, and their own feelings regarding pain, illness, and bodily physical changes. They should view aging in a positive way as a period of change, growth, and development. They should consider the elderly as a special group with a storehouse of valuable information, knowledge, wisdom, talents, and skills built up over a lifetime—as a group that can make a special contribution to society. Those who are aged 65 may live another 25 or 30 years, and it is quite possible that this final third of their lives may be the best. Keeping this fact in mind will enable the caregiver to see the importance of suicide intervention with this age group.

Zinberg (1964) has noted that psychotherapy with the elderly involves a large number of emergency situations, scheduling and transportation problems, problems of a multigenerational nature involving one or more other family members, and the coexistence of organic brain disease, psychogenic trauma, and physical illness. Those hoping to intervene successfully and prevent a geriatric suicide must be aware of and be willing to deal with such problems.

Lawton and Gottesman (1974), Gottesman (1977), Glasscote, Gudeman, and Miles (1976), and others have all noted the importance of social situations and circumstances and the physical environment as contributing factors in mental health problems of the elderly. Rather than treat only the psyche of the elderly, effective caregivers must be willing to leave their offices and work with the elderly person in the latter's home, family, neighborhood, and community. The use of existing support systems (kin, friend, church) and neighborhood resources and facilities (transportation, recreation opportunities) and involvement with family members are essential in effective intervention with the elderly.

According to Glasscote et al. (1976), three types of services are necessary to promote positive mental health in the elderly: (1) supportive services (chore services, telephone assistance, home visits, communal housing, and other services designed to keep the elderly person functioning), (2) clinical services (counseling services, geriatric day care programs, outpatient mental health services, and (3) preventive, supportive, and life-enhancing services (nutrition programs, peer support groups, legal aid, transportation, recreation programs). Gottesman (1977) suggests five roles the effective caregiver should play: (1) psychological tester (administration of various psychological tests and other instruments, such as described in Part I), (2) therapist or listener (individual and/or group psychotherapy and counseling to help the older individual cope with retirement, death of a spouse, health problems, and other problems associated with aging), (3) program developer (development of behavior modification and various other treatment programs), (4) care manager in the community (interaction with resource agencies and persons in the local community to serve the multiple needs of the elderly client), and (5) policy maker (provision and interpretation of information on various therapies and intervention strategies and on their value and impact to influence public policy).

"General health and welfare measures aimed at keeping older persons active, useful, and socially involved can undoubtedly contribute to a reduction of suicide in older people" (Busse & Pfeiffer, 1977, p. 224). Thus, in addition to the aspects discussed above, it is important to recognize the valuable role of recreation and leisure and the meaningful use of spare time in preventing suicide among the old. Until very recently, the problem with leisure was more one of finding some than of deciding how to use it. It has been only since the institutionalization of retirement, stemming from the passage of the Social Security Act in 1935, that years of leisure became a reality for large numbers in our society. Today, the elderly, described by Michelon (1954) as the "new leisure class," possess more free time, unconstrained by family and work obligations, than any other group of elderly in history, and also more than any other age group in our present society. Individuals can now expect to live about one-third of their lives in leisure. It is estimated that males can expect to have approximately 42,900 hours of leisure after retirement, based on a life expectancy of 14.0 years after age 65; and females can expect to have approximately 56,400 hours of leisure, based on a life expectancy of 18.4 years after age 65 (U.S. Senate Committee on Aging, 1981). These new hours of leisure can be a blessing—or a burden—for our elderly.

Already numerous critics have pointed to increased dehumanization, boredom, and meaninglessness in life as individuals sit idly in front of the television or engage in other leisure activities just to fill their hours and hours of "free time" (Basini, 1975; Bell, 1973; Fromm, 1955). As growing numbers of individuals live more years outside of productive employment, an increasingly important question is, How can we as a society and as practitioners working with the elderly meet the new leisure needs so that available time becomes time to be enjoyed—rather than endured?

The activity theory of aging (Lemmon, Bengtson, & Peterson, 1972; Maddox, 1963) posits a positive relationship between social activity (including leisure activity) in late life and morale or life satisfaction. Research has consistently supported this theory (De Carlo, 1974; Graney, 1975; Havighurst & Albrecht, 1953; Phillips, 1957). Those elderly individuals who remain active in groups, organizations, and social roles are the happiest in late life.

Walking, swimming, jogging, and other physical forms of exercise are a valuable form of leisure and recreation for the elderly. The physiological benefits of exercise—improved cardiovascular functioning, lowered metabolic rate, improved muscle and bone strength and flexibility, and increased physical capacity—are well documented (Cooper, 1977; Gore, 1972; Powell, 1974; Spreitzer & Snyder, 1983). Equally well documented are the psychological benefits derived from active participation in physical exercise: a natural "high," release of stress and tension through active and focused concentration on one activity without outside distraction, better mental performance and alertness resulting from the increased flow of oxygen to the brain, improved body image, a healthy vigorous feeling, and increased poise and self-confidence as a result of feeling physically in shape (Morgan, 1977; Palmore, 1979; Powell, 1974). Studies have also found that active physical exercise contributes to life satisfaction in late life (Palmore, 1979).

Kelly (1974, 1978), Neulinger (1981), Iso-Ahola (1978, 1980), and others view leisure as a state of mind. Perceived freedom and intrinsic motivation—participating just for the sheer fun or pleasure of it—are the most important elements. Released from many family and work obligations, the elderly have more discretionary time available and more chance to engage in "unconditional leisure" than those in young adulthood or middle age. The elderly may read, cook, garden, participate in drama, art or music, contemplate or reflect, build something, or engage in a hobby of particular interest. As long as the activity is freely chosen and provides a sense of pleasure and the individual is deeply involved in it, the opportunity to achieve a true "leisure state" exists. Such participation in late life provides a means of pleasure and self-satisfaction, creative expression and expansion, a sense of personal identity, and feelings of competence and mastery. It also contributes to positive self-concept and self-esteem, as well as personal development and fulfillment. All of these results are safeguards against suicide.

Apart from its expressive quality, leisure is motivated by the elderly individual's need for affiliation and social integration. Much leisure is focused on establishing or maintaining active involvements with family and friends or in the church or community (Kelly, 1978; Ward, 1979). Social forms of participation in formal and informal groups and activities can help alleviate feelings of loneliness, boredom, and despair. Such participation can also help fill the void left by lost work and lost family roles; it can provide self-esteem, personal worth, and meaning formerly derived from such work and family roles. Havighurst (1961) and Atchley (1976) suggest that leisure is a potential source of status and prestige, self-worth, and new friendships, as well as a way to be of service to others and to relieve boredom.

The effective caregiver should assume the role of leisure counselor, encouraging the lonely, depressed, or isolated elderly client to develop a hobby or physical exercise activity or to become a member in some social or recreational group in the local community. A knowledge of what is available, an awareness of the necessary skills for participation, and an understanding of the past and present interests, motivations, and physical and mental capacities of the elderly client are all essential for effective leisure counseling. In addition, the caregiver must know about locations, scheduling, transportation, cost, and other relevant details in order to encourage participation.

Techniques for Psychiatric Intervention with the Elderly

Below we offer some specific suggestions for conducting psychotherapy with the disturbed elderly, based on a review of existing literature.

- *Early detection and treatment of psychiatric disorders.* It is important for those in gatekeeping positions (doctors, nurses, social workers, ministers and pastoral staff, recreational leaders) to read accurately the signs and signals of possible suicide in the elderly. Accurate assessment of depression, loneliness, low subjective morale, and other negative feeling states may prevent a suicide. The practitioner should memorize some of the major warning signals outlined and discussed in Part I and become familiar with some of the standardized assessment tools reviewed earlier. A knowledge of recent losses or changes in environment, living conditions, or family relationships is necessary to alert the caregiver to particularly dangerous times for the elderly. Constant alertness and frequent reassessment are mandatory when dealing with suicide prevention in the elderly.

- *Adapt treatment to resources of the individual.* To intervene effectively with the elderly, the caregiver must adapt treatment to the resources that the individual possesses—the individual's physical and psychic capacities, memory, motivation, environmental factors, and support networks. A thorough knowledge of physical health and capacities, cognitive level of functioning, and living environment and existing support networks allows the practitioner to suggest appropriate interventions (group or individual, type of recreation, social, or community program, etc.). Such indepth knowledge is possible only if one takes a detailed history, administers appropriate standardized tests, meets with the family, and really gets to "know" the elderly individual.

- *An active, direct approach.* Gotestam (1980), Rechtschaffen (1959), Goldfarb (1971), and others advocate an active, direct approach with the elderly. The therapist must help define the problem and offer solutions in a strong, direct, authoritative manner. According to Goldfarb, elderly individuals should be encouraged to be dependent on the therapist, and the therapist should assume a strong authoritarian or even parental role. Often because of loss of job, health, money, or other resources, the elderly person is forced realistically into a more dependent position and needs to be accepted in the dependent state. The dependent elderly client may really want and need a rescuer, a strong person to look up to, respect, and rely upon. Unlike some other age groups, those in the older age group tend to do what they are told by doctors or other authority figures. Just telling the older person not to take all those pills may be enough to prevent a suicide.

- *A supportive attitude.* Meerloo (1961), Kastenbaum (1978), Butler (1975), and others who have successfully worked with the troubled elderly agree that loving kindness, warmth, and support are of the utmost importance when working with the aged. A friendly smile, a gentle touch, a warm accepting attitude are all therapeutic for elderly who face a hostile, ageist society that has retired and rejected them. Kastenbaum (1978) suggests creating a "therapeutic alliance" with the troubled elderly client and fostering the feeling that client and therapist are in the struggle together (p. 200).

● *Empathy.* Empathy is the ability to go beyond an objective understanding of the patient's thoughts, feelings, and behavior and to experience the world as the patient does. Unconditional positive regard and empathic understanding may be curative in and of themselves, by prompting education, retraining, or behavior modifications. Caring, empathy, and a trusting atmosphere can facilitate positive changes in elderly clients.

● *A brief, problem-centered focus.* Goldfarb (1971), Brink (1979), and others suggest that deep-insight therapy is much less appropriate for the elderly than is brief, problem-centered therapy. The latter approach may be compared to surgery in which first the problem is diagnosed, and then the surgeon gets in, solves the problem, and gets out.

● *Listening as therapy.* Butler (1975) and O'Brien, Johnson, and Miller (1979) advocate sympathetic listening as the elderly discuss their past lives or current problems and feelings. Some elderly have a great need to tell, to express feelings of guilt, fear, or doubt. For many, the caregiver may be the only person who will listen and care. Many elderly have no other interpersonal relationship except the one they share with the caregiver. Thus, for the elderly client, the caregiver is a friend and confidant as well as therapist and helper.

● *Nonverbal communication.* Butler (1975) and O'Brien et al. (1979) suggest that, because of the frequency of multiple impairment in their hearing and sight, nonverbal communication is very important in work with the aged. Burnside (1973) notes that it is important to directly face the elderly client. Tone of voice, facial expressions, nods, gestures, touches—all are important indicators of how the therapist really feels toward the elderly. The elderly can see through a facade and correctly distinguish genuine interest and concern from insincerity. The caregiver who does not really enjoy working with the aged and who does not understand their problems and losses will not be very successful.

● *Respectful treatment.* The elderly, more than any other age group, are denied the respect of others in our society, simply because they are old. They should be addressed by their full names, using appropriate titles such as Mr. or Mrs., and otherwise treated with respect. Prying or getting too personal is not tolerated by most elderly people.

- *Maintenance of coping mechanisms.* Verwoerdt (1976) correctly advises that the various defenses and coping techniques of the elderly should not be removed, which would be comparable with taking away crutches from the paralyzed. Indeed, if one defense mechanism is removed, another one is likely to take its place. The elderly often have to build up what we might consider unhealthy defenses or maladaptive coping strategies, just to survive. Clinging dependency, for example, may allow an elderly individual who would otherwise have been abandoned to survive. The task of the caregiver is to determine why particular defenses exist and then to try to encourage more adaptive coping techniques to replace less adaptive ones. The task is one of reeducating and retraining. A caring, sympathetic, empathic caregiver can effectively model appropriate behavior and teach healthier coping.

- *Objective language.* O'Brien et al. (1979) note the importance of using various objects in the environment to stimulate conversation and effect change. Reference to a cane, for example, might stimulate feelings about pain, illness, dependency, or loss. The expression of such feelings is often therapeutic.

- *Special catalysts.* Television, movies, family photos, and scrapbooks can elicit memories, feelings, or thoughts and serve as springboards for therapy with the old. Poetry, prayers, cartoons, special pictures, or favorite recipes can also serve as valuable aids to therapy with the old (O'Brien et al., 1979).

- *Goal setting.* Working with the elderly is different than working with the young. The elderly have fewer years left and have already raised their families and worked at a chosen job or career. The caregiver must have realistic expectations and goals for such individuals. With the aged, the caregiver must take a more active role in defining, setting, and helping the individual reach realistic goals. Short-term goals are more appropriate for those in the later stages of life. One major goal might be to help the elderly person adjust to a recent crisis such as death of a spouse, retirement, or a diagnosis of terminal illness. For many, an important goal might be to help them understand, accept, and adjust to the aging process. It is important to provide correct information about aging and perhaps about particular diseases so that the troubled individual knows what to expect as a "normal" condition, one that others also experience. Making the last years of life the best years might be a goal that the therapist can help the client work toward. The way to accomplish such a goal obviously will be different for each individual, and the task is to discover what each person can do to accomplish such a goal. Recommending self-help books, such as *I Can If I Want To* by Lazarus and Fay

(1975) or *The Lifelong Learner* by Gross (1977), could help some persons. For others, suggesting various support groups or recreational activities might be more effective. Some might choose to compile their life histories or write their life stories before they die. One goal of therapy with elderly individuals is to assist them in accomplishing the developmental tasks of late life. Coming to terms with death—their own and that of their loved ones—and achieving a sense of ego integrity (Erikson, 1950), a sense that their life has been meaningful and worthy of having been lived, are two major developmental tasks of late life. A final therapeutic goal might be to help elderly individuals actualize their potential as creative human beings. However, a thorough knowledge of the individual's interests, talents, skills, and limitations is necessary before this goal can be reached.

INTERVENTION WITH THE "AT-RISK" ELDERLY

The elderly individual who shows signs of severe depression or displays clues of possible suicide must be identified and helped. As we have already pointed out, elderly individuals rarely attempt incomplete suicide; rather they carry through and kill themselves—all the more reason why early detection and appropriate intervention are crucial with this group.

The caregiver who is armed with an adequate understanding of the signs and symptoms of depression and suicidal risk and who has a genuine love, concern, and respect for the elderly and the problems of growing old should become familiar with and be able to handle nine critical areas in dealing with suicidal individuals (Hatton, Valente, McBride, & Rink, 1977):

1. building trust and rapport
2. dealing with one's own feelings of professional inadequacy
3. overcoming one's fear of responsibility for making decisions that might in fact encourage suicide in the client
4. coming to terms with suicidal feelings or impulses in one's self
5. handling special resentment of the client
6. avoiding subjective comparisons of the client with one's self or with other individuals
7. handling listening difficulties so that one is able to listen empathically
8. really focusing on the individual's problem
9. avoiding stereotyping of the individual

In order to intervene effectively with a suicidal older individual, it is important to establish a trusting, caring relationship in which the individual feels comfortable, accepted, supported, and loved. It is important to build trust, respect, and a sense of mutuality between caregiver and client. It is essential for the helping agent to question the person directly regarding the person's thoughts about, or actual plans for committing, suicide. Many elderly suicides could be prevented if someone merely asked the individuals simply and directly if they were contemplating suicide and then let them talk. It is crucial to *listen, listen, listen* to the older person. Sometimes the messages are subtle; often the real feelings are transmitted through nonverbal communications. Thus direct questioning about suicidal intent must be handled correctly. Hatton et al. (1977) provide the following examples of proper and improper questions (pp. 68–69):

Improper	*Proper*
You're *not* suicidal, are you???	You've been feeling so miserable, I wonder if you have considered suicide?
Oh, come on (jokingly), you aren't really suicidal!	I would like to hear more about your suicidal feelings.
You say you're suicidal, but I want to know what is *really* bothering you.	Please tell me about any suicidal thoughts or feelings you may have.
	I'm concerned that you may be feeling suicidal. Are you feeling suicidal now?

Once suicidal intent has been clearly established, the following steps in intervention are suggested (Hatton et al., 1977, pp. 73–76):

- *Focus on the current hazard or crisis.* The caregiver needs to help the disturbed individual focus on the worst problems and gain a clear perspective on them.
- *Reduce any immediate danger.* If the individual has pills available clearly direct that they not be taken, using a direct statement such as, "I want you to flush the pills down the toilet." Have the person promise not to try to commit suicide before the next meeting.
- *Evaluate the need for medication.* When the danger of suicide is imminent, antidepressants may be required.
- *Evaluate the need for someone to be present.* If it appears that the person is in imminent danger of self-destruction, a family member, friend, neighbor, or significant other should be asked to stay with the person.
- *Mobilize the client's internal and external resources.* Success in reducing suicide may depend on getting the individual reinvolved in the family, friendships, neighborhood, or community or on reorienting the individual and mobilizing internal coping mechanisms for survival. The individual may need to be helped to structure a day or a week of time.

The caregiver may have to find activities, support systems, transportation, and other resources for the individual. Finally, the teaching of new problem-solving techniques might be necessary.

• *Implement a plan of action.* Effective intervention must help the troubled elderly reverse their thinking and direction. An ongoing structured program of help must be planned. It is important to involve family, friends, and neighborhood and community agencies in this stage in intervention.

All of these steps in intervention are appropriate for the at-risk elderly. Above all, the caregiver who works with elderly clients should keep in mind that these individuals are "special" in the sense that they face real losses in physical and mental capacity, financial losses, losses of family and friends, and loss of love and respect as individuals.

REFERENCES

Abrahams, R., & Patterson, R. D. (1978). Psychological distress among the community elderly: Prevalence, characteristics, and implications for service. *International Journal of Aging and Human Development, 9,* 1–18.

Atchley, R. C. (1976). *The sociology of retirement.* New York: John Wiley & Sons.

Basini, A. (1975). Education for leisure: A sociological critique. In J. T. Haworth & M. A. Smith (Eds.), *Work and Leisure* (pp. 102–117). London: Lepus Books.

Bell, D. (1973). The coming of post-industrial society. New York: Basic Books.

Berg, R. L., Browning, F. E., Hill, J. G., & Wenkert, W. (1970). Assessing the health care needs of the aged. *Health Services Research, 3,* 36–59.

Brill, N. W., & Storrow, H. A. (1960). Social class and psychiatric treatment. *Archives of General Psychiatry, 3,* 36–59.

Brink, T. (1979). *Geriatric Psychotherapy.* New York: Human Sciences Press.

Burnside, I. (1973). Long-term group work with hospitalized aged. In I. Burnside (Ed.), *Psychosocial nursing care of the aged* (pp. 202–214). New York: McGraw-Hill.

Busse, E. W., & Pfeiffer, E. (1977). *Behavior and adaptation in late life.* Boston: Little, Brown & Co.

Butler, R. (1975). *Why survive? Being old in America.* New York: Harper & Row.

Butler, R., & Lewis, M. (1977). *Aging and mental health.* St. Louis, Mo.: C. V. Mosby.

Cooper, K. H. (1977). *The aerobic way.* New York: M. Evans.

De Carlo, T. J. (1974). Recreation participation patterns and successful aging. *Journal of Gerontology, 29,* 416–422.

Erikson, E. (1950). *Childhood and society.* New York: W. W. Norton.

Fromm, E. (1955). *The sane society.* New York: Holt, Rinehart & Winston.

Gaitz, M. (1974). Barriers to the delivery of psychiatric services to the elderly. *Gerontologist, 14,* 3.

Glasscote, R., Gudeman, J. E., & Miles, C. D. (1976). *Creative mental health services for the elderly.* Washington, D.C.: American Psychiatric Association.

Goldfarb, A. (1971). Group therapy with the old and aged. In H. Kaplan & B. J. Sadock (Eds.), *Comprehensive group psychotherapy* (pp. 623–642). Baltimore, Md.: Williams & Wilkins.

Gore, I. Y. (1972). Physical activity and aging—A survey of Soviet literature, I. Some of the underlying concepts. *Gerontology Clinician, 14,* 65–69.

Gotestam, K. G. (1980). Behavioral and dynamic psychotherapy with the elderly. In J. E. Birren & R. B. Sloane (Eds.), *Handbook of mental health and aging* (pp. 775–805). Englewood Cliffs, N.J.: Prentice-Hall.

Gottesman, L. E. (1977). Clinical psychology and aging: A role model. In W. D. Gentry (Ed.), *A model of training and clinical service* (pp. 1–7). Cambridge, Mass.: Ballinger.

Graney, M. (1975). Happiness and social participation in aging. *Journal of Gerontology, 30,* 701–706.

Gross, R. (1977). *The lifelong learner.* New York: Simon & Schuster.

Group for the Advancement of Psychiatry, Committee on Aging, (1971). *The aged and community mental health: A guide to program development* (Vol. 8, Series 81). New York: Author.

Hamburg, D. A., Bibring, G., Fisher, C., Stanton, A. H., Wallerstein, R.S., Weinstock, H.I., & Haggard, E. (1967). Report of the ad hoc committee of the American Psychoanalytic Association cited for gathering data. *Journal of the American Psychoanalytic Association, 15,* 841–861.

Hatton, C. L., Valente, S., McBride, S., & Rink, A. (Eds.). (1977). *Suicide: Assessment and intervention.* New York: Appleton-Century-Crofts.

Havighurst, R. J. (1961). The nature and value of meaningful freetime activity. In R. W. Kleemeir (Ed.), *Aging and leisure* (pp. 309–344). New York: Oxford University Press.

Havighurst, R. J., & Albrecht, R. (1953). *Older People.* Green, N.Y.: Longmans.

Hollingshead, A. B., & Redlich, F. C. (1958). *Social class and mental illness.* New York: John Wiley & Sons.

Iso-Ahola, S. E. (October, 1978). *The social psychology of leisure and recreation.* Paper presented at the NRPA research symposium, Miami, Fla.

Iso-Ahola, S. E. (1980). *The social psychology of leisure and recreation.* Dubuque, Iowa: William C. Brown.

Kahn, R. L. (1975). The mental health system and the future aged. *Gerontologist, 15,* 24–31.

Kastenbaum, R. (1964). The reluctant therapist. In R. Kastenbaum (Ed.), *New thoughts on old age* (pp. 139–145). New York: Springer.

Kastenbaum, R. (1978). Personality theory, therapeutic approaches, and the elderly. In M. Storandt, I. Siegler, & M. Elias (Eds.), *The clinical psychology of aging* (pp. 199–225). New York: Plenum Press.

Kelly, J. R. (1974). Socialization toward leisure: A developmental approach. *Journal of Leisure Research, 6,* 181–193.

Kelly, J. R. (1978). Situational and social factors in leisure choices. *Pacific Sociological Review, 21,* 313–330.

Knight, R. (1978–1979). Psychotherapy and behavior change with the noninstitutionalized aged. *International Journal of Aging and Human Development, 9,* 221.

Lawton, M. P., & Gottesman, L. E. (1974). Psychological services to the aged. *American Psychologist, 29,* 689–693.

Lazarus, A., & Fay, A. (1975). *I can if I want to.* New York: Warner Books.

Le Bray, P. E. (1979). Geropsychology in long-term care settings. *Professional Psychology, 10,* 474–484.

Lemmon, B. V., Bengtson, V. L., & Peterson, J. A. (1972). An exploration of the activity theory of aging: Activity types and life satisfaction among in-movers to a retirement community. *Journal of Gerontology, 27,* 511–523.

Lowenthal, M. F., Berkman, P., Brissette, G. G., Buehler, J. A., Pierce, R. C., Robinson, B. C., & Trier, M. L. (1967). *Aging and mental disorder in San Francisco.* San Francisco: Jossey-Bass.

Maddox, G. (1963). Activity and morale: A longitudinal study of selected elderly subjects. *Social Forces, 42,* 195–204.

Meerloo, J. A. M. (1961). Geriatric psychotherapy. *Acta Psychotherapeutica, 9,* 169–182.

Michelon, L. C. (1954). The new leisure class. *American Journal of Sociology, 59,* 371–378.

Morgan, W. P. (1977). Involvement in vigorous physical activity with special reference to adherence. *Proceedings of the National College of Physical Education Association for Men,* 235–246.

Neulinger, J. (1981). *To leisure: An introduction.* Boston: Allyn & Bacon.

O'Brien, C., Johnson, J., & Miller, B. (1979). Counseling the aging: Some practical considerations. *Personnel and Guidance Journal,* 288–291.

Palmore, E. B. (1979). Predictors of successful aging. *Gerontologist, 19,* 427–431.

Phillips, B. S. (1957). A role theory approach to adjustment in old age. *American Sociological Review, 22,* 212–217.

Powell, R. R. (1974). Psychological effects of exercise therapy upon institutionalized geriatric mental patients. *Journal of Gerontology, 29,* 157–161.

Rechtschaffen, A. (1959). Psychotherapy with geriatric patients: A review of the literature. *Journal of Gerontology, 14,* 73–84.

Schaffer, L., & Myers, J. (1954). Psychotherapy and social stratification. *Psychiatry, 17,* 83–89.

Schofield, W. (1964). *Psychotherapy: The purchase of friendship.* Englewood Cliffs, N.J.: Prentice-Hall.

Smith, C. (1979). Use of drugs in the aged. *Johns Hopkins Medical Journal, 145,* 61–64.

Sparacino, J. (1978–1979). Individual psychotherapy with the aged: A selective review. *International Journal of Aging and Human Development, 9,* 197–200.

Spreitzer, E., & Snyder, E. E. (1983). Correlates of adult participation in adult recreation sports. *Journal of Leisure Research, 15,* 27–38.

Storandt, M., Siegler, I., & Elias, M. (Eds.). (1978). *The clinical psychology of aging.* New York: Plenum Press.

U. S. Senate Committee on Aging. (1981). *Developments in aging: 1980 (Pt. 1).* Washington, D.C.: U.S. Government Printing Office.

Verwoerdt, A. (1976). *Clinical geropsychiatry.* Baltimore, Md.: Williams & Wilkins.

Ward, R. (1979). *The aging experience.* New York: Lippincott.

Zinberg, N. E. (1964). Geriatric psychiatry: Need and problems. *Gerontologist, 4,* 130–135.

Chapter 6

Pharmacological Interventions

Soo Borson and Richard C. Veith

The value of drugs in the treatment of psychiatric disorders rests on their ability to alter deranged physiological patterns. Affective disorders (depression and mania), schizophrenia, alcohol intoxication and withdrawal, anxiety disorders, and certain states of demoralization are all characterized by abnormal biological as well as psychological functioning. The development of techniques to measure neurotransmitters, hormones originating in and acting on the brain, electrical activity of the brain's various parts, and brain structure (as visualized by computed axial tomography, positron emission tomography, and nuclear magnetic resonance) has permitted rapid growth of biological psychiatry within the past two decades.

Depression, the most thoroughly studied of the major psychiatric disorders to date, is, in a significant proportion of patients, associated with measurable disturbances in urine, plasma, and cerebrospinal fluid (CSF) levels of norepinephrine and its metabolites, regulation of cortisol secretion by the adrenals, and neuroendocrine responses to pharmacologic challenge (see Sachar, Asnis, Halbreich, Nathan, & Halpern, 1980, for a detailed summary of current knowledge).

Several recent reports suggest that there may be a unique biologic substrate for suicidal behavior that is distinguishable from that of the underlying illness. Reported abnormalities in suicide attempters with either depression or personality disorders (Brown, Ebert, & Goyer, 1982; Meltzer et al., 1984; Traksman, Asberg, Bertilsson, & Sjostrand (1981) include persistent failure to normalize the function of the hypothalamic-pituitary-adrenal axis after

Soo Borson, M.D., is Assistant Professor, Department of Psychiatry and Behavioral Sciences, School of Medicine, University of Washington, Seattle, Washington. Richard C. Veith, M.D., is Associate Professor, Department of Psychiatry and Behavioral Sciences, School of Medicine, University of Washington, and Clinical Investigator, Geriatric Research, Education and Clinical Center, Seattle-American Lake Veterans Administration Medical Center, Seattle, Washington.

apparently successful treatment of depression (Targum, Rosen, & Capodanno, 1983), low ratio of urinary norepinephrine to epinephrine in conjunction with high urinary cortisol excretion (Ostroff et al., 1982), and low levels of 5-hydroxyindoleacetic acid (a metabolite of the neurotransmitter serotonin) in cerebrospinal fluid. These findings may eventually provide a rational basis for therapeutic trials of drugs targeted specifically at violent self-destructive behavior.

In this chapter, we review the role of drugs in the management of the psychiatric disorders that predispose to suicide among the elderly, touch on the indications for electroconvulsive treatment (ECT), and discuss the place of individual psychotherapeutic approaches as adjuncts to pharmacotherapy. We stress that drug therapy is not without hazard, particularly in older patients; age-related pharmacokinetic changes tend to prolong the action of many drugs, increase the risk of adverse effects due to unwanted accumulation of drugs in the body, and set the stage for multiple drug interactions with potentially serious outcome (Vestal, 1978). In addition, changes in brain receptors for drug action may be altered with aging, increasing sensitivity to a given dose of drug (Vestal, 1982). As a consequence, greater caution, lower starting doses, and slower incremental changes are required in treating older as compared to younger persons. Attention to coexisting medical illness—especially involving the heart, liver, kidneys, or brain—and simplification of drug regimens when possible will help ensure safe, effective use of psychotropic drugs. In general, the minimum effective course of treatment, combined with suitable, adjunctive nonpharmacologic treatments, is most desirable.

AFFECTIVE DISORDERS

Major depression is a clinical syndrome characterized by despondency, emotional pain, or physical complaints that are out of proportion to existing disease and fail to respond to reassurance; reduced capacity to experience pleasure; withdrawal of interest in others; and alteration of vital functions and biological rhythms (activity, energy, concentration, appetite, and sleep). This syndrome is believed to underlie at least two thirds of suicides in the elderly (Gurland & Cross, 1983). Most elderly suicides have been depressed less than a year (Barraclough, 1971), often developing their illness after bereavement (MacMahon & Pugh, 1965), the onset of an acute or serious chronic disease (Kay, Beamish, & Roth, 1964), or a change of residence required by circumstances (Sainsbury, 1973).

Depressive illnesses, while sharing core diagnostic features, differ widely in their clinical presentations. Pictures most likely to be associated with suicidal outcome in the elderly are the severe, agitated, hypochondriacal, panic-ridden, "involutional" depressions with marked insomnia, self-neglect, and confusional episodes (Barraclough, Bunch, Nelson, & Sainsbury, 1974), and delusional depressions, diagnosed as unipolar, bipolar, or schizo-affective types. Chronic, milder depressive states—which limit adaptation to stressors such as losses, interpersonal conflict, financial strain, and illness—can set the stage for certain suicides, but no reliable data are available on this point. However, it is suggested by the findings of two studies (Barraclough, 1971; Miller, 1978) that the majority of elderly suicides are outpatients who have seen their primary doctor within three months of death, received some psychotropic drug (usually not an antidepressant), suffered from long-term sleep disturbance (suggesting depression), and were not referred to any specialist in mental health care.

There is compelling evidence that different clinical subtypes of depression require different pharmacologic strategies. The spectrum of agents useful in the treatment of affective illness in the aged includes tricyclic antidepressants, monoamine oxidase inhibitors (MAOIs), newer nontricyclic agents, lithium, neuroleptics, sedative-anxiolytics, and central stimulants. These represent essentially the entire pharmacopoeia for treatment of mental disorders; therefore, their use in nonaffective conditions, where relevant, is reviewed here as well. Thereafter, we present a brief account of nonpharmacologic approaches to depressive disorders, including ECT and certain defined psychotherapeutic interventions for which research data are available.

Drugs

Tricyclic Antidepressants

Approximately nine tricyclic agents are currently available. They are most useful in the treatment of depressions characterized by pervasive dysphoria or persistent and widespread loss of interest associated with the typical endogenous symptom pattern (gradual onset, prominent anhedonia, distur-bances of sleep, appetite, and psychomotor activity) (Bielski & Friedel, 1976). They sometimes can produce dramatic benefits, however, in carefully selected chronic depressives whose symptoms are more intermittent and less pervasive (Cassano, Maggini, & Akiskai, 1983).

Tricyclic antidepressants are thought to act on central monoamine pathways, particularly at noradrenergic and serotonergic sites, to facilitate synaptic transmission. Agents differ in their relative selectivity for the two aminergic systems, hence failure of treatment with one does not always imply failure with a second. Choice of antidepressant is currently based on relative differences in side effect profiles. Veith (1982) offers a clinically practical discussion of this issue, including dosage guidelines, use of plasma drug levels in assessing adequacy of treatment, adverse effects and contraindications, drug interactions, and duration of treatment.

Monoamine Oxidase Inhibitors

Three agents—phenelzine, tranylcypromine, and isocarboxazid—are available for use at present. MAOIs block monoamine oxidase, an enzyme widely distributed in both the central nervous system and peripherally; and optimal drug response requires at least 80 percent inhibition of this enzyme. MAOIs appear to have particular value in younger anxious, irritable, and "atypical" lethargic depressions and certain depressed bipolar patients. They may produce marked clinical improvement in patients of any age who are unresponsive to tricyclics. The clinical profile of geriatric depressives not responsive to these agents is unclear. Therefore, MAOIs should rarely be the drug of first choice, unless a patient is known to be intolerant of, or refractory to, tricyclics.

The main side effects of MAOIs are predictable from their inhibitory effects on breakdown of serotonin, dopamine, and norepinephrine. They include sedation or insomnia, movement disorders, altered bladder function, hypotension, and potential for serious interactions with sympathomimetic and certain other drugs ("Monoamine Oxidase," 1980). MAOIs also inhibit the degradation of tyramine, produced from the amino acid tyrosine during fermentation of foods. Hypertension, bronchial constriction, headache, and coronary vasoconstriction can occur when aged foods are eaten by persons taking MAOIs. Stroke and myocardial infarctions can occur in patients with preexisting vascular insufficiency. However, when dietary and drug precautions are followed, these agents are often better tolerated by elderly persons than are tricyclics. Effective doses range from 7.5 mg of phenelzine, or equivalent, to 60–90 mg, with lower doses generally effective for the older person.

Newer Nontricyclic Agents

Maprotiline

A tetracyclic agent, maprotiline displays a pharmacologic profile similar to imipramine. It has mild to moderate sedative and moderate anticholinergic side effects and appears to offer no clear advantage over imipramine, which is less expensive.

Bupropion

Bupropion is expected to be marketed in the United States in the near future. It represents a new class of effective antidepressants whose mechanism of action is unknown (Ferris, Cooper, & Maxwell, 1983). Because of its relative lack of reported anticholinergic and cardiovascular side effects (Wenger & Stern, 1983), it is expected to find wide acceptance in the treatment of geriatric depression; clinical trials with elderly depressed patients have been promising (Branconnier et al., 1983; Kane, Cole, Sarantakos, Howard, & Borenstein, 1983). As for all new drugs with which clinical experience is limited, faddish overprescribing is to be avoided.

Lithium

The main indications for lithium use in elderly patients are bipolar affective illness with acute mania and affective cycles occurring more often than every three years. Recognition of bipolar illness or its variants, the schizo-affective psychoses of late life, may be difficult when confusion, dementiform symptoms, or paranoia are prominent in a hyperactive, agitated patient; a history of earlier episodes may be lacking. Because lithium is our most effective drug for long-term management of these psychotic illnesses, accurate diagnosis is critical. Occasionally, patients with true dementia (Alzheimer's disease, multiinfarct dementia, or others) develop endogenous mania-like syndromes and may benefit from lithium.

The clinical use of lithium in the elderly presents certain challenges. Aging narrows the range between therapeutic and toxic doses, and coexisting medical problems must be carefully monitored (Veith, 1984). Side effects may involve any organ system; of special concern are insidiously developing hypothyroidism, cardiac sinus node dysfunction, and clinically important interaction with diuretics. Because plasma lithium clearance is directly dependent upon renal function, which is normally reduced with aging, required doses are often smaller in elderly patients than in younger patients. Doses of lithium may be as low as 50 mg/day to start, with 150–300 mg/day more usual. Dose increments every three to four days to achieve a serum level of 0.4–0.7 mEq/L are usually adequate (Roose, Bone, Haidorfer, Dunner, & Fieve, 1979). Decisions about long-term lithium maintenance treatment must be individualized, weighing the risks of toxic effects against those of recurring manic decompensation.

Neuroleptics

Neuroleptics, the mainstay of drug management in acute and chronic schizophrenia, are used in the treatment of acute mania and in depressive illness characterized by delusions or marked confusion and disorientation. Major depression with delusions responds better to combined treatment with antidepressants and neuroleptics than to antidepressants alone (Glassman, Kantor, & Shostak, 1975; Nelson & Bowers, 1978). However, combining drugs in the elderly compounds the risk of side effects, which may require discontinuation of treatment and institution of ECT.

Particularly troublesome side effects of the neuroleptics in older patients are loss of motor speed and precision, large muscle weakness and/or stiffness or Parkinson rigidity (especially with the lower-dose agents such as haloperidol), and falls due to orthostatic hypotension (especially with the high-dose agents such as chlorpromazine). Other less common but equally important side effects are reviewed by Veith (1984).

Sedatives/Anxiolytics

Depressed patients with marked agitation or insomnia may benefit from a brief course of sedatives early in their treatment, since the tricyclics require three to six weeks or more for full antidepressant effect. Sedatives can dull depressive misery, keeping the patient more comfortable during this expected lag time. In practice, however, most patients experience significant relief of anxiety and insomnia during the first week of antidepressant therapy, requiring no additional classes of drugs. When an anxiolytic is needed, oxazepam may be preferable to diazepam, chlordiazepoxide, or lorazepam because of its briefer half-life and absence of active metabolites. Doses of 10–30 mg up to four times a day may be given; lower doses less often are preferable, if effective.

The use of long-term benzodiazepine treatment for chronic anxiety states has been controversial. Recent evidence suggests that the risk of habituation and tolerance has been overrated (Rosenbaum, 1982), but drug interactions and subtle (or not so subtle) motor and cognitive effects must be anticipated by the clinician prescribing for the elderly.

Hypnotics have definite value in management of short-term sleep problems associated with hospitalization, bereavement, and other acute life disruptions. However, about a third of older patients report unsatisfactory sleep, often for long periods. Before reaching for the prescription pad, the clinician must develop a working grasp of the problem: age-related changes in sleep pattern, medical or psychiatric disorders, chronic unresolved tensions, and insecurity at night—particularly among the frail elderly living alone who may never relax their vigilance enough to sleep well—all require their own approach. Attention to underlying causes of sleep complaints can save the clinician time in the long run by improving specificity of treatment and also demonstrate concern for what is, to the patient, a greatly distressing symptom. When a hypnotic is called for, a short-acting agent—such as triazolam, which has been shown to have minimal daytime carryover in mental and motor performance in elderly patients—is probably safer (Ayd, 1983).

Central Stimulants

Dextroamphetamine and methylphenidate have clinical value in certain apathetic, older patients; in patients with depression who cannot tolerate tricyclics and are not impaired enough to warrant ECT; and, as enhancers of tricyclic action, in patients with partial responses to tricyclics. They are well-tolerated by most patients in doses of 5–20 mg/day, but the specific antidepressant agents are more effective. With development of new classes of antidepressants with demonstrated efficacy, the place of stimulants is likely to be further restricted. For withdrawn nursing home patients, stimulants have not been shown to be superior to environmental stimulation.

Nonpharmacologic Treatment Modalities

Electroconvulsive Therapy

ECT is the single most effective intervention for serious late-life depression; and, despite public controversy over its use in recent years, it has been demonstrated to be safe when applied according to established guidelines (Kendell, 1981). Even patients with serious medical disorders accompanying affective illness maybe treated with relatively low risk and high benefit (Bidder, 1981). Concern over the possibility of lasting brain damage due to ECT has been excessive. The data indicate that memory loss with ECT is almost always transient and far less disabling than the cognitive deficits due to untreated severe depression (Malloy, Small, Miller, Milstein, & Stout, 1982).

Psychotherapy

Many styles of individual psychotherapy have been used in the treatment of older patients with mild mood disorders, crises of adjustment, problem behavior, and family difficulties. The clinical literature on psychotherapy is large and does not lend itself to generalization, except to emphasize that an understanding, supportive relationship with a skilled therapist clearly fosters both comfort and behavior change for many troubled elders. The recent interest in psychogeriatrics, the growth of training programs, and the increase in the number of relevant professional publications are helping to make this kind of relationship more available to those who can benefit from it.

Results of the first prospective trial of the efficacy of psychotherapy for depression in the elderly have been reported by Gallagher and Thompson (1983). They compared brief cognitive, behavioral, and insight-oriented supportive therapies in randomly assigned elderly outpatients with nonendogenous ("neurotic" mood depression) and endogenous depressive episodes (with disturbed sleep, activity, interest, and appetite, as well as mood). The results indicated that brief cognitive and behavioral therapies are effective in nonendogenous depression and superior to a brief supportive approach. They are not effective against endogenous depression, and trials of combined pharmacotherapy and psychotherapy are presently underway elsewhere.

ANXIETY DISORDERS

Certain forms of early-onset, recurring anxiety disorders are associated with increased long-term suicide risk (Coryell, Noyes, & Clancy, 1982). Although a disposition to "neurotic" anxiety and compulsive, rigid personality traits have long been recognized as antecedents to late-life depression and therefore may contribute to certain suicides, we do not yet have studies relating geriatric suicide to the primary, "endogenous" anxiety disorders now recognized as distinct psychobiologic entities in the American Psychiatric Association's *Diagnostic and Statistical Manual of Mental Disorders*, third edition (DSM III) (American Psychiatric Association, 1980). Generalized anxiety disorder, panic disorder, and obsessive-compulsive disorder—the three main primary anxiety states—have not been studied systematically in the elderly with respect to prevalence, natural history, or treatment. Because of the high frequency of anxiety symptoms seen among elderly persons in all health care settings, we summarize below current knowledge of their forms and management.

Anxiety and Restlessness

Anxiety states and restlessness occur frequently in association with late-life depressive illnesses. Sometimes the most visible symptoms, they may obscure the underlying affective disorder and its proper treatment. Anxiety as a symptom of affective illness responds well to antidepressant treatment, rarely requiring separate consideration. Clinically anxious, nondepressed patients must be carefully evaluated for medical causes of distress (especially cardiorespiratory disease), drug-induced states, and early dementing illness. When treatable medical causes of anxiety have been attended to, patients with persistent anxiety should be managed from an interdisciplinary perspective, emphasizing remediable sources of loss of security and training in relaxation techniques, supplemented with small doses of sedatives (benzodiazepines or antihistamines) if needed. Drugs tend to become ineffective over time if the sources of anxiety persist. Chronic anxiety probably predisposes to late-onset alcoholism, sedative habituation, cental nervous system toxicity (particularly cognitive and motor), and polypharmacy when the physician misses the anxiety underlying the patient's shifting complaints. Occasionally, chronically anxious nondepressed patients respond to low doses of tricyclic antidepressants (e.g., imipramine 10–25 mg/day).

Panic States

Panic states are common in individuals with late-life affective psychoses and in patients who have recently survived potentially fatal episodes of disease, particularly myocardial infarction. Impulsive suicide is a clear risk in these situations, as panic dissolves the capacity to evaluate one's situation realistically while causing unbearable discomfort. Neuroleptics are usually the drugs of choice, because of their rapid onset of action and potent calming effects; antidepressants or lithium are added as appropriate for associated depressive or mixed manic-depressive illness, and ECT may be used for rapid termination of a dangerous panic. In nonaffective patients whose panic follows overwhelming illness, supportive psychotherapy—involving help in understanding their emotional responses, in enhancing their physical and emotional supports in day-to-day life, in helping to restore their self-esteem, and in preparing for death—is necessary once panic has abated with drugs. Consider the following case:

A 77-year-old retired contractor with a 10-year history of serious ischemic heart disease sustained a massive near-fatal myocardial infarction, requiring resuscitation and maximum life support. During recovery, he experienced escalating anxiety, which failed to respond to larger and larger doses of benzodiazepines and evolved into a drug-induced delirium. The full picture of a manic psychosis appeared as sedatives were withdrawn—with pressured, loud speech, flight of ideas, physical intrusiveness and threats, sleeplessness, and suicidal and homicidal ideas. Haloperidol 5 mg twice a day completely suppressed the symptoms and was stopped after four days, leaving him coherent and aware of the sources of his massive anxiety. After six weeks of psychotherapy in the hospital, he returned home with fluctuating but manageable levels of anxiety, off drugs. He knew that his life would soon end, but he had largely mastered his terror of death that had set the stage for his anxiety psychosis. He died relatively peacefully of heart failure three months later.

Syndromes resembling separation anxiety as seen in children may occur in the impaired elderly and prompt suicidal ideation or attempts. These syndromes are not well delineated in the geriatric age group; however, studies in children and in phobic-avoidant anxious adults demonstrate the differential efficacy of tricyclic antidepressants over anxiolytics. For example:

> A man aged 87, mildly mentally deficient since birth but independent in adulthood, developed heart block requiring the insertion of a cardiac pacemaker. Following surgery, he made daily suicide threats and attempted to jump out the window. Psychiatric examination showed long-term intellectual deficits with no memory loss, pervasive dysphoria, or vegetative signs of depression. Every day around 4–5 P.M., he began to hover about the nurses, complaining of feeling upset and unwilling to let them out of his sight. His suicidal ideation abated as his emotional attachments grew; nortriptyline 10 mg. daily abolished his anxiety and clinging behavior completely.

Obsessive-Compulsive Disorders

Phobic illness and obsessive-compulsive disorders may result in a homebound, irrationally fearful, rigidly structured personality that intensifies with age and impoverishes life. Clinical depression is a risk. Pharmacotherapy has not been tried systematically for these anxiety-related syndromes in the elderly; experience suggests that drugs (especially the tricyclics or MAOIs) are likely to be effective in acute cases but are less likely to be accepted, or to help, in longstanding disorders that have become interwoven with personality.

ALCOHOLISM

Chronic Alcoholism

Late-onset alcoholism is associated with risk for suicide attempts in 5 to 20 percent of drinkers over age 60 (Schuckit & Pastor, 1978). No drug, other than disulfiram (Antabuse), has demonstrated value in the management of chronic alcoholism per se (Halikas, 1983). Disulfiram acts as an aversive conditioning agent by interacting with imbibed alcohol to produce a characteristic reaction, consisting of facial flushing, cough, difficulty in breathing, anxiety, vomiting, and elevated blood pressure. It therefore tends to limit impulsive drinking. The alcohol-disulfiram reaction is potentially fatal in patients with serious liver, cardiovascular, and cerebrovascular disease, in persons with moderate to severe diabetes mellitus or cognitive impairment, and in the frail elderly. Disulfiram interacts with certain other prescribed drugs (e.g., hypnotics, anticoagulants, and diphenylhydantoin), and its reaction with alcohol may be enhanced by antidepressants and antihypertensives. These facts dictate that the use of disulfiram to promote abstinence in the elderly alcoholic should be considered only after careful, complete medical evaluation and systematic appraisal of risks.

Schuckit (1982) has outlined the general approach to treatment of the elderly alcoholic. Elements include identification of the problem, confrontation with the facts, recommendation of abstinence, recruitment of family members or others in the patient's everyday environment, legal action (e.g., alcohol commitment) if warranted, and close attention to coordinating the multiple medical, social, and recreational services important in long-term rehabilitation. Schuckit stresses the centrality of helping such patients to reorganize their daily lives without alcohol and of addressing the psychological issues common to the development phase of late adulthood—decline in social and physical potency, decline in relations with adult children and spouse, loneliness, boredom, and lack of purpose. An effective course of treatment is likely to take a year, with gradually decreasing intensity as normal routines are restored.

Acute Alcohol Intoxication and Withdrawal

The seriously intoxicated elderly person with medical illness and/or behavioral disturbances requires protective intervention to end the alcoholic episode and manage its potentially dangerous complications. This often implies hospitalization for supportive care, detection of such alcohol-related medical problems as gastrointestinal bleeding and pneumonia, and management of withdrawal. Pharmacologic treatment of withdrawal states is aimed at substituting a safer central nervous system depressant for alcohol, gradually tapering the dose as signs and symptoms of withdrawal abate. Benzodiazepines remain the drugs of choice for this purpose, with chlordiazepoxide still most widely used. Dosage determination is empirical, with the goals of suppressing the acute anxiety, confusion (delirium), and autonomic hyperactivity (tachycardia, sweating, nausea, vomiting, diarrhea, and blood pressure changes of the withdrawal state). Fatalities still do occur from delirium tremens; older patients require special vigilance to prevent dehydration and cardiovascular collapse.

A reasonable approach to drug treatment of alcohol withdrawal in the older patient is to begin with chlordiazepoxide 25–50 mg orally, then to monitor the effects on symptom severity and vital signs hourly and repeat the dose upon reappearance of symptoms and signs of withdrawal. If liver disease is suspected, a better choice of drug might be oxazepam 20–60 mg, since this drug yields no active metabolites to accumulate and produce unexpected oversedation later on. Once a dose schedule adequate to suppress symptoms without excessive sedation is established, daily reduction of 10–20 percent should permit detoxification within five to seven days. Mild anxiety and depression, tremor, sleep disturbance, and minor autonomic instability are common in long-term alcoholics for months to years after discontinuation of drinking and should be treated nonpharmacologically whenever possible. Drug interventions should be limited to reliably abstinent patients with symptoms severe enough to interfere with their daily lives; in these cases, a psychiatric diagnosis other than alcoholism is usually warranted.

Secondary Alcoholism

Secondary alcoholism is alcoholism that develops in the course of a defined psychiatric disorder, usually as a response to symptoms (anxiety, tension, irritability, confusion, unbearable depression, psychotic terror, or manic excitement). Alcohol tends to worsen the symptoms in the long run and adds its own characteristic disabilities. Prognosis for treatment is that of the primary condition (Halikas, 1983), and appropriate treatment is likely to diminish the drinking behavior. It is unclear whether late-onset alcoholism is more likely to be symptomatic of another psychiatric illness, such as depression, than early-onset alcoholism, but it is clear that both primary and secondary alcoholism may develop at any age. A scrupulous search for underlying depressive illness, atypical schizoaffective psychoses, and panic or demoralization related to failure to recover from losses can yield great rewards in the older alcoholic who comes for treatment for the first time. Consider the following two cases:

A 68-year-old retired logger and lifelong social drinker was brought by his wife for hospitalization when he began to drink heavily, drive his truck wildly about the hills, and pester a neighbor for sexual favors. Two hospitalizations and a serious suicide attempt occurred before the presence of a late-onset, cyclic, schizoaffective psychosis was recognized. ECT, followed by lithium maintenance, terminated the psychosis and the excessive drinking.

An 82-year-old retired, highly successful mechanical engineer was hospitalized after threatening his wife of 60 years with a knife, menacing the staff, and attempting suicide three times in the nursing home where he was placed by his son for his increasing "senility." His moderate drinking began five years earlier. Heavy drinking began one year earlier when his 54-year-old, bachelor son was fired from his job and "retired" to his bedroom in the family home, sleeping by day and carousing with friends at night. Six months later, the patient was hospitalized with a bleeding duodenal ulcer and cirrhosis of the liver. No attempt was made to treat his alcoholism; the unusual and conflicted relations between the son, wife, and patient were not noted. On admission, the patient demonstrated a florid toxic psychosis with a negative blood alcohol level. All symptoms disappeared when several medically prescribed drugs were withdrawn, leaving the patient in a state of painful awareness of the tragic effect his illness had had on his family and himself. Upon detailed testing after three weeks, no evidence of any mental disorder was detected, other than some forgetfulness too mild to impair day-to-day function. No clear-cut psychiatric disorder preceded his increased drinking, which he attributed to boredom, to unresolved friction with his wife over their never-emancipated, middle-aged son, and to his own failing health and hearing. Family therapy in the hospital convinced the wife to drop guardianship proceedings. A hearing aid improved his participation in conversation and decreased his feelings of isolation. Family-oriented treatment for alcoholism was recommended. Special issues to be addressed included the triadic enmeshment of the family, the spouses' habitual estrangement despite continuing love for each other, and the son's pathologic dependence on the father at a time when the latter needed more support himself.

DEMORALIZATION STATES

Severe, lasting demoralization is most likely to be encountered in older persons suffering from seriously and chronically disabling medical illness. The daily toll of such illness on vitality, stamina, appetite, restful sleep, and body appearance produces gradual but progressive shrinkage of the life space, with diminishing opportunities for stimulation, healthy intimacy, and the exercise of personal competence. With increasing physical dependency, interpersonal relationships gradually shift toward the instrumental. Active attempts to commit suicide in this group of patients are unusual, but quiet decisions to relinquish a life grown too burdensome are not. Ethical conflicts involving the patient's right to die versus the doctor's obligation to treat may complicate the situation.

Specific psychopharmacologic interventions offer little in the management of this kind of demoralization. Such patients do, however, develop identifiable depressive episodes (often heralded by a medically unexplained deterioration of physical function, by increased dependency, or by personality change) that respond to treatment like other depressive episodes. When apathy seems out of proportion to the degree of illness but the full depressive syndrome is lacking, amphetamines or methylphenidate may stimulate interest and improve the patient's mood, with relatively little risk of adverse effects.

The tools of the general physician, rehabilitation specialist, social worker, financial counselor, and clergy may substantially improve the sick, demoralized patient's ability to tolerate severe impairment with equanimity; such tools are the mainstays of management.

REFERENCES

American Psychiatric Association. (1980): *Diagnostic and statistical manual of mental disorders* (3rd ed.). Washington, D.C.: Author.

Ayd, F. J. (1983). Triazolam. *International Drug Therapy Newsletter, 18*(1), 1–4.

Barraclough, B. M. (1971). Suicide in the elderly. In D. W. K. Kay & A. Walk (Eds.), *Recent developments in psychogeriatrics* (pp. 87–97). Ashford-Kent, England: Hedley Brothers.

Barraclough, B., Bunch, J., Nelson, B., & Sainsbury, P. (1974). One hundred cases of suicide. *British Journal of Psychiatry, 125*, 355–373.

Bidder, T. G. (1981). Electroconvulsive therapy in the medically ill patient. *Psychiatric Clinics North America, 4*, 391–406.

Bielski, R. J., & Friedel, R. O. (1976). Prediction of tricyclic antidepressant response: A critical review. *Archives of General Psychiatry, 33*, 1479–1489.

Branconnier, R. J., Cole, J. O., Ghazvinian, S., Spera, K. F., Oxenkrug, G. F., & Bass, J. L. (1983). Clinical pharmacology of bupropion and imipramine in elderly depressives. *Journal of Clinical Psychiatry, 44*(5:2), 130–133.

Brown, G. L., Ebert, M. H., & Goyer, P. F. (1982). Aggression, suicide, and serotonin: Relationships to CSF amine metabolites. *American Journal of Psychiatry, 139*, 741–746.

Cassano, G. B., Maggini, C., & Akiskai, H. S. (1983). Short-term, subchronic, and chronic sequelae of affective disorders. *Psychiatric Clinics North America, 6*, 55–68.

Coryell, W., Noyes, R., & Clancy, J. (1982). Excess mortality in panic disorder: A comparison with primary unipolar depression. *Archives of General Psychiatry, 39*, 701–703.

Ferris, R. M., Cooper, B. R., & Maxwell, R. A. (1983). Studies of bupropion's mechanism of antidepressant activity. *Journal of Clinical Psychiatry, 44*(5:2), 74–78.

Gallagher, D. E., & Thompson, L. W. (1983). Effectiveness of psychotherapy for both endogenous and nonendogenous depression in older adult outpatients. *Journal of Gerontology, 38*, 707–712.

Glassman, A. H., Kantor, S. J., & Shostak, M. (1975). Depression, delusions, and drug responses. *American Journal of Psychiatry, 132*, 716–719.

Gurland, B. J., & Cross, P. S. (1983). Suicide among the elderly. In M. K. Aronson, R. Bennett, & B. J. Gurland (Eds.), *The acting-out elderly* (pp. 55–65). New York: Haworth Press.

Halikas, J. A. (1983). Psychotropic medication used in the treatment of alcoholism. *Hospital and Community Psychiatry, 34*, 1035–1039.

Kane, J. M., Cole, K., Sarantakos, S., Howard, A., & Borenstein, M. (1983). Safety and efficacy of bupropion in elderly patients. *Journal of Clinical Psychiatry, 44*(5:2), 134–136.

Kay, D. W. K., Beamish, P., & Roth, M. (1964). Old age mental disorders in Newcastle-upon-Tyne. Part II: A study of possible social and medical causes. *British Journal of Psychiatry, 110*, 668–682.

Kendell, R. E. (1981). The present status of electroconvulsive treatment. *British Journal of Psychiatry, 139,* 265–283.

MacMahon, B., Pugh, T. F. (1965). Suicide in the widowed. *American Journal of Epidemiology, 81,* 23–31.

Malloy, F. W., Small, I. F., Miller, M. J., Milstein, V., & Stout, J. R. (1982). Changes in neuropsychological test performance after electroconvulsive therapy. *Biological Psychiatry, 17,* 61–67.

Meltzer, H. Y., Umberkoman-Wita, B., Robertson, A., Tricou, B. J., Lowy, M., & Perline, R. (1984). Effect of S-hydroxytryptophan on serum cortisol levels in major affective disorders. II: Relation to suicide, psychosis, and depressive symptoms. *Archives of General Psychiatry, 41,* 379–387.

Miller, M. (1978). Geriatric suicide: The Arizona study. *Gerontologist, 18,* 488–495.

Monoamine oxidase inhibitors for depression. *Medical Letter.* (1980). *22,* 58–60.

Nelson, J. C., & Bowers, M. D. (1978). Delusional unipolar depression. *Archives of General Psychiatry, 35,* 1321–1328.

Ostroff, R., Gillen, E., Bonese, K., Ebersole, E., Harkness, L., & Mason, J. (1982). Neuroendocrine risk for suicidal behavior. *American Journal of Psychiatry, 139,* 1323–1325.

Roose, S. P., Bone, S., Haidorfer, C., Dunner, D. L., & Fieve, R. R. (1979). Lithium treatment in older patients. *American Journal of Psychiatry, 136,* 843–844.

Rosenbaum, J. F. (1982). The drug treatment of anxiety. *New England Journal of Medicine, 306,* 401–404.

Sachar, E. J., Asnis, G., Halbreich, V., Nathan, R. S., & Halpern, F. (1980). Recent studies in the neuroendocrinology of major depressive disorders. *Psychiatric Clinics North America, 3,* 313–326.

Sainsbury, P. (1973). Suicide: Opinion and facts. *Proceedings of the Royal Society of Medicine, 66,* 579–587.

Schuckit, M. A. (1982). A clinical review of alcohol, alcoholism, and the elderly. *Journal of Clinical Psychiatry, 43,* 396–399.

Schuckit, M. A., & Pastor, P. A. (1978). The elderly as a unique population: Alcoholism. *Alcoholism: Clinical and Experimental Research, 2,* 31–38.

Targum, S., Rosen, L., & Capodanno, A. E. (1983). The dexamethasone test in suicidal patients with unipolar depression. *American Journal of Psychiatry, 140,* 877–879.

Traksman, L., Asberg, M., Bertilsson, L., & Sjostrand, L. (1981). Monoamine metabolites in CSF and suicidal behavior. *Archives of General Psychiatry, 38,* 631–636.

Veith, R. C. (1982). Depression in the elderly: Pharmacologic considerations in treatment. *Journal of the American Geriatrics Society, 30,* 581–586.

Veith, R. C. (1984). Treatment of psychiatric disorders. In R. E. Vestal (Ed.), *Drug treatment in the elderly* (pp. 317–337). Sydney, Australia: ADIS Health Science Press.

Vestal, R. E. (1978). Drug use in the elderly: A review of problems and special considerations. *Drugs, 16,* 358–382.

Vestal, R. E. (1982). Pharmacology and aging. *Journal of the American Geriatrics Society, 30,* 191–200.

Wenger, T. L., & Stern, W. C. (1983). The cardiovascular profile of bupropion. *Journal of Clinical Psychiatry, 44*(5:2), 176–182.

Chapter 7

Support Groups

HISTORICAL OVERVIEW

From the beginning of recorded history, human groups have been used as healing agents, as exemplified by the primitive tribal rituals and war dances of cave men and the classical Greek chorus.

Prior to 1900, both the hypnotist Anton Mesmer and the infamous Marquis de Sade, who used mental patients as actors in theatrical productions, practiced group therapy. However, it was not until the twentieth century that medical and mental health professionals recognized the curative powers of groups and began to use them in therapeutic intervention. J. H. Pratt first employed group methods effectively with tuberculosis patients in 1907. In 1925, J. L. Moreno developed a method of group therapy called psychodrama. In the 1940s, World War II created a situation in which the needs for psychiatric intervention far outstripped the available mental health resources. Thus, the use of group therapy expanded greatly out of both necessity and experience. Since World War II, group therapy has gained wide use as a curative process.

Group therapy or group counseling applied as an intervention strategy for the elderly is a more recent phenomenon. There are several reasons why group therapy has only recently been adopted for use with the elderly. First, the Freudian approach not only denigrated group therapy in general, it particularly emphasized the futility of psychotherapy for people in later stages of life. Second, many health professionals avoided working with the elderly. They believed many of the myths and stereotypes about aging and the elderly. They did not believe the elderly talk enough and they did not regard them as good candidates for therapy; or they were prejudiced against the elderly and felt they were not worth their time and trouble because, after all,

"They don't have much time left anyway, so why bother?" or they had not themselves successfully faced and dealt with the issues of aging and their own deaths. In short, many health professionals were "reluctant therapists" (Kastenbaum, 1964, p. 139) when it came to dealing with the aged.

Third, the elderly themselves tended to resist group therapeutic help, particularly when it was offered by mental health professionals. To seek help was to admit weakness and was viewed as a stigma by many elderly individuals. Kramer, Taube, and 'Redick (1973), Eisdorfer and Stotsky (1977), Hendricks and Hendricks (1977), and Zarit (1980) noted the reluctance of elders to use mental health services, primarily because of their negative perceptions of mental health work.

The first references to group psychotherapy with the elderly appeared in 1950. Silver (1950) was the first to use group psychotherapy successfully with the elderly; his patients were senile psychotics. In 1956, Linden, another pioneer in the field, successfully employed group therapy with the institutionalized aged. Subsequently, Wolff (1957, 1963), Benaim (1957) and Stein (1959) used group psychotherapy effectively with the institutionalized elderly.

During the 1950s and into the 1960s, most group work with the aged was a form of psychotherapy conducted in institutions. Over time, those working with the elderly in groups gradually began to shift their emphasis from psychoanalytic personality and insight therapy to more problem-oriented, discussion types of therapy. Reminiscence and emphasis on daily living concerns were seen as more appropriate for this age group and replaced personality change and insight as the major focus.

In the 1960s, although most group work with the elderly was still focused on the institutionalized, some outpatient and community group work began to appear. Social workers and nurses used group work effectively with the elderly (Burnside, 1969, 1971, 1978; Kubie & Landau, 1953; Lucas, 1964; National Association of Social Workers, 1961/1980; Yalom & Terrazas, 1968). However, at this point it was difficult to distinguish therapy groups from discussion or social activity groups, and most group work combined all three elements.

Since the late 1960s, group work with the aged has blossomed. A variety of professionals—social workers, nurses, psychiatrists, psychologists, and recreation leaders—are effectively using many different kinds of groups in a variety of settings, including nursing homes, age-segregated communities, private outpatient programs, housing projects, and other community settings.

VARIETIES AND VALUES OF GROUP WORK

Freud insisted that "the number of patients was of no psychological significance and thus . . . there was no need to develop new concepts to explain the phenomena which occur in group psychotherapy" (Horton & Linden, 1982, p. 55). He saw the group as just a set of individuals that could be perceived solely in terms of individual psychodynamics: "Group psychotherapy is seen as individual psychotherapy in a group setting" (Horton & Linden, 1982, p. 55). The Freudian perspective thus promoted individual psychotherapy as the sole method of treatment. Similarly, others see two important advantages of individual psychotherapy compared to group work: (1) greater attention to individual problems on a one-to-one basis and (2) achievement of deeper insight (Knight, 1979; Ronch & Maizler, 1977). Indeed, Kastenbaum (1966) has demonstrated the effectiveness of individual counseling with the older adult.

More recently, influenced by the postulate of gestalt psychology that the whole is more than the sum of its parts, practitioners and researchers alike have cited the numerous benefits of group work, particularly with the elderly. Linden (1956) has noted that "it is the unusual event in medicine to find a single therapeutic agent that recommends itself as appropriately, offers supplies for as many needs, and manages the total person as felicitously as does group psychotherapy in the relief of the emotional disorders of later years" (p. 129). In fact, a review of the literature suggests that one's sense of alienation is reduced and one's social functioning is enhanced when interacting with others in a group (Lieberman, Yalom, & Miles, 1973). In outlining the many benefits of group work—that is, "all programs in which small face-to-face groupings are utilized to promote socializations, better interpersonal relationships, improve role behavior and task performance, and rehabilitation"—Scheidlinger noted that "far-reaching therapeutic effects can occur in the sickest of people through group influence measures considerably removed from what one would consider as psychotherapy" (Ross, 1975, p. 508).

Bednar and Kaul (1978) and Kaul and Bednar (1978) identify four factors which distinguish group therapy from individual therapy: In a group, the members (1) learn by their participation in developing and evaluating a social microcosm, (2) learn by giving and receiving feedback, (3) have the unique opportunity to be both helpers and helpees, and (4) learn by the consensual validation of multiple perspectives. As a counseling method, group work has several advantages over individual therapy. As noted by Yalom (1970) and Burnside (1978), the group offers opportunities for people to confront feelings of alienation by providing for free expression of feelings and experiences with group members who are "in the same boat." It also provides a vehicle for members to learn from one another and to share information, experiences, and hints on problem solving. It offers a place to learn and practice interpersonal skills that enhance friendships and family relationships. Finally, it can instill hope in members who see others successfully coping with similar problems or life experiences (Yalom, 1970).

Because of the social aspect of group therapy, opportunities to give and receive feedback are plentiful. As members are faced with a variety of different behaviors, personalities, and histories, they see many subjective realities, and come to choose their reality based upon their own selves as referents (Kaul & Bednar, 1978). In whatever form it takes, feedback appears to be a basic human need—to find out how one is seen by others, and also how one sees other individuals. Many clients seen in therapy have low self-esteem and poor self-concepts, which are often detriments to helping others. However, participation in group counseling often results in a reciprocal relationship of helping and being helped.

No matter what type of group one is participating in, there appears to be some degree of mutual sharing. An atmosphere of acceptance and under-standing is essential for such sharing to occur. Often, the discovery of similarities is extremely therapeutic. With the sharing of emotional feelings and experiences, individual members begin to have a sense of communion, and a sense of belonging develops that has often been lacking in their individual lives. Also, the sense of safety the group offers provides members with support, caring, friendship, and encouragement.

Group therapy can be defined as "the use of group methods and activities to encourage personal activity, sociability, and social integration of the group member" (Goldfarb, 1972, p. 113). As we have noted, this type of therapy is particularly appropriate for the elderly. The emotional and physical disabilities of the elderly are often due to precipitating life stresses, not the irreversible process of old age (S. R. Saul & S. Saul, 1974). Indeed, it is now generally accepted that many of the elderly's dysfunctions are social in nature rather than the result of chronological aging. In his study in a geriatric state mental hospital, Benaim (1957) concluded that a primary need of old people is a social need and that group psychotherapy thus becomes a most effective means of treatment. His program involved a once-a-week directive therapy group centered on family problems, loneliness, and neglect—all common ailments of the aged. For many of the participants, the group provided their only source of social contact.

Lieberman, Yalom, and Miles (1973) suggest that social isolation and loneliness can be effectively reduced through participation in group work. Lowy (1967) notes that group counseling provides the adult with opportunities to learn and practice new social roles to replace lost roles. Group interaction allows older adults to discuss problems and concerns regarding the new roles. Group work with the elderly also serves to enhance a positive "cohort effect" (Burnside, 1978), as members discover that they share a common history and future and similar interests, concerns, and problems.

Participation in groups offers the elderly a way to pass the hours and meet and socialize with new friends. They can regain control over their lives through the sharing of information and insights and involvement with role models who have successfully faced the same problems. As Verwoerdt (1976) notes, "Supportive psychotherapy with aged patients is best carried out in a group context. The experience in the group enhances a sense of belonging, also an appreciation for the value of external sources of satisfaction, and effectiveness of reality testing" (p. 138). In such a context, a group intervention can avoid some of the pitfalls of individual therapy with the elderly, such as ineffective counseling due to the counselor's own unresolved feelings toward aging and death, countertransference by counselors who inappropriately assign an elderly client the role of parent and react on that basis, and the detrimental effects of age bias on the counseling relationship (Mardoyan & Weiss, 1981).

TYPES OF SUPPORT GROUPS

A variety of groups have been used by nurses, social workers, psychiatrists, and laymen in nursing homes, day care centers, churches, and other community settings. Capuzzi and Gross (1980) distinguish four types of groups that may benefit the elderly:

1. Reality orientation groups, which assist individuals who are experiencing disorientation with respect to time, place, people, or things. Such groups reorient the participants toward reality through various sensory exercises and the use of television and other pragmatic techniques.
2. Reminiscence groups, which utilize life reviews, autobiographies, and personal remembering of past events, people, and places to help the participants achieve ego integrity and deal with aging and death.
3. Remotivation groups, which are designed to motivate and stimulate an active interest in life in those who are apathetic and depressed.
4. Psychotherapy groups, which are clinically oriented groups designed to allow expression of fears, anxieties, doubt, guilt, and other emotions and to bring unconscious thoughts, feelings, and emotions to the surface where they can be acknowledged, expressed, and dealt with by the individual. Art, music, dance, and drama therapy groups fall in this category.

Activity and recreational groups and clubs have been used to provide the elderly with social exchanges and interaction and meaningful leisure time and to offer creative outlets and mechanisms to achieve self-esteem, personal mastery, status, prestige, and social integration (Atchley, 1976; Havighurst, 1961; Kaplan, 1953; Shore, 1964). More specialized groups—variously referred to as member-specific groups, special topic groups, theme groups, mutual help groups, or self-help groups—have recently provided popular and effective coping mechanisms for many elderly, particularly those experiencing a crisis or transition state. All of these types of groups can aid in implementing effective intervention strategies for the lonely, isolated, or depressed elderly who are facing crises of terminal illness, coping with the loss of a loved one, or trying to deal with the multiple losses of aging.

CHARACTERISTICS OF SUPPORT GROUPS

Caplan defines support systems as "continuing social aggregates (namely, continuing interactions with another individual, a network, a group, or an organization) that provide individuals with opportunities for feedback about themselves and for validation of their expectations about others, which may offset deficiencies in these communications within the larger context" (Caplan & Killilea, 1976, p. 19). Caplan has linked this definition with the work of Cassel (1974), which demonstrated a lower incidence of mental and physical disease among those involved in such networks compared with those who were not. Kahn and Antonucci (1979) cite many studies that show that such support systems moderate the effects of stress and disease. Caplan (1974) suggests that the major reason for this is that each member of the support system is dealt with as a unique individual.

> The other people are interested in him in a personalized way. They speak his language. They tell him what is expected of him and guide him in what to do. They watch what he does and they judge his performance. They let him know how well he has done. They reward him for success and punish or support and comfort him if he fails. Above all, they are sensitive to his personal needs, which they deem worthy of respect and satisfaction.

> Such support may be of a continuing nature or intermittent and short-term and may be utilized from time to time by the individual in the event of an acute need or crisis. Both enduring and short-term supports are likely to consist of three elements: (a) the significant others help the individual mobilize his psychological resources and master his emotional burdens; (b) they share his tasks; and (c) they provide him with extra supplies of money,

materials, tools, skills, and cognitive guidance to improve his handling of his situation. (Caplan, 1976, pp. 19–20)

Others have defined a support system as "that set of personal contacts through which the individual maintains his social identity and receives emotional support, material aid, services, information, and new social contacts" (Campbell & Chenoweth, 1980, p. 3). The major role of the family in providing this type of support has been well documented (Lowenthal & Robinson, 1976; Sussman, 1976). However, groups with nonkin members can also serve as supportive networks (Pilsuk & Minkler, 1980).

As a support system, the family functions as a collector and disseminator of information, a feedback guidance system, a source of ideology, a guide and mediator in problem solving, a source of mutual aid, a haven for rest and recuperation, a reference and control group, a source and validator of identity, and a place for emotional expression (Caplan, 1976). Many of these functions also characterize other types of support or mutual help groups. Self-help groups like Alcoholics Anonymous and Gamblers Anonymous and peer support groups like those for grievers who have lost a spouse provide what Vickers (1971) calls "an appreciative system sufficiently widely shared to mediate communications, sufficiently apt to guide action, and sufficiently acceptable to make personal experience bearable" (p. 439).

Kropotkin (1914/1925) suggested that human evolution has been possible only through mutual aid, the joining together and helping of one another to struggle in common against the forces of nature. This principle of mutual aid or joint struggle against common problems underlies the development of mutual help or support groups. The attachments formed in such groups:

> serve to improve adaptive competence in dealing with short-term crises and life transitions as well as long-term challenges, stresses and privations through (a) promoting emotional mastery, (b) offering guidance regarding the field of relevant forces involved in expectable problems and methods of dealing with them, and (c) providing feedback about an individual's behavior that validates his conception of his own identity and fosters improved performance based on adequate self-evaluation. (Caplan, 1974, p. 2)

Phyllis Silverman, noted for her efforts in starting the Widow-to-Widow Program, defines mutual help groups as:

> those organizations that limit their membership to individuals with common problems. The purpose of such organizations is to help the members and others with the same difficulties solve their mutual

problems. In time, recipients of help will move to become helpers. Solutions offered usually have specific and concrete applications for solving problems; help can go both ways, and is usually offered in a personal and informal fashion. Most often such groupings develop around critical transitions in a person's life, when other solutions are unavailable or ineffective. In a mutual help group, the individual is not defined as deviant or as a patient, but as someone undergoing a natural and normal experience, such as bereavement or childbirth. (Silverman & Cooperband, 1975, pp. 13–14)

Support groups are particularly effective for individuals facing situational stress or distress, that is, "reactions that are so much the product of exposure to a particular situation that they are displayed by almost everyone in the situation" (Weiss, 1976, p. 213). For example, typical responses to the loss of a spouse are depression, restlessness, loneliness, loss of appetite, fatigue, and irrational or impulsive behavior. Weiss (1976) defines three such situations in which support in the form of understanding, accepting, and caring is particularly important: (1) a crisis situation, a very sudden, traumatic upset of relatively short duration that results in a persistent disruption of the former state of equilibrium; (2) a transition state, a period of relational and personal change usually necessitated by some crisis; and (3) a deficit situation, a state in which some important element—such as love, money, or health—is unobtainable, thus necessitating creation of a new life structure.

Those in these kinds of situations are vulnerable to stress, disease, emotional breakdown or illness, even suicide, and are in great need of supportive help. Those in a transition state are particularly open to receive help. Such individuals are confused and upset and are searching for information, answers, and supportive relationships. Specifically, as noted by Weiss (1976), individuals who are in transition are subject to obsessive review; anger, guilt, and related emotions; uncertainty regarding self; a tendency to false starts; impulsive moves and mistakes; and self-doubt or lack of self-confidence. Involvement in a support group can help in resolving such problems.

Support groups are patterned after the family or small community and are expressive in nature. They offer members understanding and acceptance as unique personalities with both good and bad qualities, with both strengths and weaknesses. They offer a place where emotions can be freely expressed and where recognition, status, and security are offered. Most support groups are established by and for individuals who are stigmatized, either for a short time or permanently (Traunstein & Steinman, 1973). For example, widows may feel they are "misfits," "marginals," or "fifth wheels" in a couple-oriented society. The very word, widow, has negative connotations and carries a stigma for many women. Those who have had an ostomy or mastectomy operation may also feel stigmatized. In a support group, these individuals can find acceptance among others suffering the same plight. When everyone shares the same stigma, one finds acceptance, and feelings of isolation and marginality are reduced. Such a group can also serve as a mediating structure (Mizruchi, 1964), softening the negative blows of the larger culture.

Several other beneficial characteristics of support groups have been identified in the literature by Caplan and Killilea (1976). Such groups can provide:

- *A common sharing of problems.* Katz (1972), Silverman (1970, 1975), Pomeroy (1972), and others cite the fact that members share a common problem as the basis of mutuality and sharing. The caregiver and receiver share the same problem; someone who has "been there before" is often the only person who can be an effective change agent.

- *Mutual help and support.* Support groups meet on a regular basis and offer mutual aid and emotional support to members on a continuing, nonconditional basis.

- *Exchange of help.* Support groups allow one to give as well as receive help. Often the opportunity to give help or care for another is as therapeutic to the helper as to the one being helped. The one being helped also later has the opportunity to provide help and service to another.

- *Socialization to new ideas, roles, and behaviors.* Often those who most need and can most benefit from support groups are those who have lost valuable social roles, meaningful relationships, mobility, or a physical part of the self. Such individuals can learn appropriate behaviors and roles from others who serve as role models and teachers in the group. The elderly particularly benefit from what Irving Rosow (1967) calls "concomitant socialization."

- *Collective will power and belief.* Frank (1973) notes that the major benefits of such groups stem from the fact that the members look to each other to validate feelings and attitudes.

- *Information and education.* Support groups are a valuable source of information, both factual and in terms of coping and problem solving. Silverman and Cooperband (1975) note the importance of providing information on such subjects as finance, legal matters, and housing, as well as concrete advice on how to cope with loneliness and depression, raising children alone, and other problems stemming from the loss of a spouse.

Table 7-1 presents a comparison of 20 characteristics of orthodox psychotherapy with those of therapy in one form of support group, the self-help group.

TECHNIQUES AND CASE ILLUSTRATIONS

Support groups are widely used today as effective intervention mechanisms with the elderly. They are helping the elderly cope with almost all of the losses and developmental crises of aging, particularly chronic illness, death or illness of a spouse, and various negative changes accompanying the aging process.

Illness and Death

There is a positive relationship between old age, dying, and bereavement. There is nothing pleasant about facing death, and it is for this reason that problems often arise in such situations in individualized counseling. A "conspiracy of silence" often results from such one-on-one therapy (Franzino, Geren, & Meiman, 1976, p. 44). In a study of the interactions of a group approach to break this silence, it was observed that the group process assisted women with a diagnosis of terminal cancer in adjusting to their impending death (Franzino et al., 1976).

As one ages, physical limitations and dysfunctions are likely to emerge. Groups are useful in helping members cope with necessary medical procedures, such as becoming bound to a wheelchair or living with an artificial limb. Acceptance of physical limitations and learning to adapt to chronic conditions resulting from such illnesses as cancer, lung disease, heart attack, and stroke have been successfully accomplished through group therapy and discussion.

Support groups also help the well spouse cope with problems related to the illness. Often it is the well spouse who provides physical care and emotional support on a 24-hour basis, sometimes to the point of physical and emotional exhaustion, who needs the most help and support. In addition, confusion, fear, anxiety, and guilt are all experienced by the caregiving spouse. In such situations, support groups can provide valuable information on the illness, proper care, and financial and legal matters. Such groups can also offer the well spouse a safe place for emotional expression and acceptance.

One of the early pioneers in group therapy with the elderly, Pratt (1907), worked with patients suffering from tuberculosis. Pratt believed that the provision of information and emotional support in a small group could speed recovery. He organized "classes" for his tuberculosis patients; the patients received visits from a friendly visitor, often a nurse, who provided instruction

Table 7-1 A Comparison of Orthodox Psychotherapy and Self-Help Group Therapy

Orthodox Psychotherapy	*Self-Help Group Therapy*
1. Professional, authoritative therapist.	Nonprofessional leaders; group parity.
2. Fee.	Free.
3. Appointments and records.	None.
4. Therapy-oriented milieu (psychiatrist's office, clinic, etc.).	Nontherapy oriented milieu (church rooms, community centers, etc.).
5. No family confrontation.	Family encouraged.
6. Psychiatrist is presumed normal, does not identify with patient.	Peers are similarly afflicted, identify with each other.
7. Therapist is not a role model, does not set personal examples.	Peers are role models, must set examples for each other.
8. Therapist is noncritical, nonjudgmental, neutral and listens.	Peers are active, judgmental, supportive, critical and talk.
9. Patients unilaterally divulge to therapists; disclosures are secret.	Peers divulge to each other; disclosures are shared.
10. Patients expect only to receive support.	Patients must also give support.
11. Concerned about symptom substitution if underlying causes are not removed.	Urges appropriate behavior; not concerned about symptom substitute.
12. Accepts disruptive behavior and sick role, absolves patient, blames cause.	Rejects disruptive behavior and sick role, holds member responsible.
13. Therapist does not aim to reach patient at "gut level."	Peers aim to reach each other at "gut level."
14. Emphasis on etiology, insight.	Emphasis on faith, willpower, self-control.
15. Patient's improvement is randomly achieved.	Patient's behavior is planfully achieved.
16. Therapist-patient relationship has little direct community impact.	Peers' intersocial involvement has considerable community impact.
17. Everyday problems subordinated to long-range cure.	Primary emphasis on day-to-day victories: another day without liquor or drugs, another day without panic, etc.
18. Extracurricular contact and socialization with psychiatrist discouraged.	Continuing support and socialization available.
19. Lower cumulative dropout percentage.	Higher dropout percentage.
20. Patient cannot achieve parity with psychiatrist.	Members themselves become active therapists.

Source: From *Support Systems and Mutual Help: Multidisciplinary Explorations* (pp. 65–66) by G. Caplan and M. Killilea (Eds.), 1976, New York: Grune & Stratton. Copyright 1976 by Grune & Stratton. Reprinted by permission.

as well as personal support. Patients also met together in Dr. Pratt's office in small groups once a week to share information, to hear personal testimony from those who were progressing well, and to provide inspiration and emotional support.

Barton (1962) reported favorable results from work with older hospitalized patients who met in a seniors veterans group. Barton attributed the favorable adjustment of the elderly participants to the group experience that assisted them in universalizing their problems, developing their skills through education, and increasing their feelings of self-respect and self-worth through mutual exchange, interaction, and acceptance. Rosin (1975) similarly employed support groups as therapeutic tools in a chronic disease hospital. Discussion groups focused on psychological problems of the physically ill, such as depression, loss of hope, disappointment, and problems in doctor-patient relationships. The group discussion was found to decrease tension and conflict and increase catharsis and interpersonal relationships.

Group work has proven to be particularly effective with elderly diabetics and arthritics. Schwartz and Goodman (1952) reported on the effectiveness of group therapy with 19 diabetic patients, most of whom were elderly. The groups were primarily educational and information-sharing groups conducted by a medical doctor. As a result of participation in the groups over a period of 18 months, the patients experienced feelings of identification with the group in relation to common problems, a strengthening of the relationship of the individual to the group leader, increased education about the problem, and a sense of group member competition.

Petty, Moeller, and Campbell (1976) organized support groups for elderly arthritics. Four groups, ranging in size from six to nine members, were composed of individuals who were 52 to 85 years of age and suffering from arthritis. Most of the individuals were experiencing moderate depression in adjusting to the aging process. Support groups were organized as informal workshops to provide a nonthreatening atmosphere for sharing. The groups met 10 times in two-hour sessions. Some common themes that emerged in the group sessions concerned depression, social isolation, and adjustment to sensory and health losses. Pretests and posttests were administered to the members in order to determine the direction and extent of change on various physical and mental health indicators. Data analysis revealed that participation in a support group decreased feelings of loneliness, depression, and unhappiness, increased knowledge of physical functioning, and resulted in better communication with family and friends and a desire to be more actively involved in life. The members also came to feel that their frustration and problems were "normal" and a part of aging. They made new friends and learned how to use community resources more effectively through their participation in the group.

Cancer is particularly prevalent among older individuals; and it probably creates more fear and dread among such individuals than any other illness. Not only must older cancer patients face their own personal fears and anxieties about pain and death, they also often experience painful operations and treatments, loss of body parts, and unpleasant, mutilating physical changes. Support groups offer a very effective therapeutic strategy for those afflicted with cancer. Such groups allow them to gather valuable information on their condition, on various medical procedures and prostheses, and on dealing with the medical establishment.

Support groups are a ready source of other persons with similar problems or stigmas who are coping successfully. Reach to Recovery, a mutual help organization of women who have had mastectomies, I Can Cope, another mutual help group for cancer patients, and other such groups are available to cancer patients throughout the country. Lenneberg and Rowbotham (1970) report on the benefits of support groups for ileostomy patients:

> Necessity drove patients to consult one another for advice on keeping one's self clean and functioning in daily pursuits . . . . It was very quickly obvious to surgeons that their patients were not only learning a great deal from mutual exchange on practical matters, they also seemed no longer to feel alone and therefore were less unhappy with their new "plumbing" . . . . At his first group meeting he will see that not only his model has solved the problems, others have also achieved success. From the group he learns further attitudes with regard to specific problems, and he gets group know-how. Professional speakers come and educate him; the appliance chairman gives him information; he is in ileostomy school.
>
> Access to such a model promotes the visualization of the self with the condition, and when the model has been successful, positive identification can take place in the patient. Conversely, if the model has not been successful, negative identification may be established, or the model may not be accepted. This mechanism of the psyche, which happens in all human situations, is the root of mutual aid between troubled and previously troubled people. (pp. 81–84)

Such support groups are also available to coronary patients and those suffering from other common debilitating diseases.

Problems of the Caring Spouse

Support groups have also been shown to be effective for spouses of ill husbands or wives. Beaulieu and Karpinski (1981) recognized the need for support for the elderly with ill spouses, couples who experience a changed marital relationship as one spouse becomes a patient and the other a caretaker. They organized support groups for the caretakers of ill spouses, the "nonidentified clients." It was felt that group treatment would "address the issue of isolation and be helpful because older people require peer support to sustain their ego image and self-confidence and to anchor them in times of swift transition and social discrimination" (p. 552). The groups emphasized psychological support as a way to encourage attitudes that allow for better functioning and ability to cope and a way to build up compensatory strengths. Each group was comprised of two men and four women. The groups met for 12 weeks. As the group members discussed their mutual problems of loneliness and isolation, decisions about institutionalizing a sick spouse, and problems of dealing with the medical establishment and with friends and relatives, they became like a caring family. After meeting in such support groups, the caretakers felt better and had a reduced sense of crisis. Many found meaningful ways to fill their time.

Alzheimer's disease is a devastating affliction that affects those in midlife or late life. The personal deterioration that results from this condition and the serious financial problems that it causes for the family are well recognized by professionals. Support groups for family members of Alzheimer's disease victims have sprung up all over the country. Work by Harkins and Wentzel in Richmond, Virginia, demonstrates that such groups provide an effective arena for information sharing, emotional expression, love, and caring.

Stichman and Schoenberg (1972) describe a support program for wives of coronary patients. The program employs counselors to help women going through the crisis. These "heart-wife" counselors are "women who have been through it helping women who are going through it" (p. 156). In describing the program, Stichman and Schoenberg report that:

> the wife is eager for reassurance; a woman whose husband recovered from the same illness is made to order. "Recovery" is the kind of talk she wants to hear. And the counselor offers a special kind of empathy she can't get even from her family. It is heartfelt; more important, it is knowledgeable. What the counselor is really saying to the wife is, "I know what you're going through, I know just what it feels like; I have been there, too." Soon the wife has the relief of letting go, letting herself say the words she was afraid to

say, expressing the thoughts she was trying desperately not to think. She has a safety valve.

During the crisis phase, the heart-wife counselor also provides a role model, gives anticipatory guidance about what's coming next, and offers concrete assistance with problems that must be dealt with immediately, such as placing calls to other members of the family, providing for care of children, and making arrangements about the patient's employment or business. In the meantime, the psychologist is working with the patient in a program of crisis intervention to ameliorate the psychological sequelae of a sudden severe illness. In Phase II, through joint meetings with professionals, other wives of hospitalized cardiac patients in the same boat, and the heart-wife counselors who have successfully been through the experience, the emphasis moves from emergency help with immediate problems and reassurance to education, preparation for homecoming, and problem-solving. Throughout the phases, the heart-wife counselors are available by telephone at any time. In Phase III, after homecoming, the program continues with monthly mutual help meetings of ex-patients and their wives, with other members of the family joining from time to time. The meetings give the families a chance to compare notes on what adjustment problems have come up and explore ways of handling them . . . . They offer a chance for full, frank discussion among people who share the same basic problem and who, therefore, understand each other's problem as no outsider could. (Caplan & Killilea, 1976, pp. 50–51)

Loss of a Spouse

A particularly traumatic life crisis that many elderly experience is the loss of a spouse. Such a loss is perhaps one of the cruelest of life's injuries. As noted earlier, those who have lost a spouse are especially vulnerable to loneliness, depression, despair, and suicide. Holmes and Rahe (1967) identify the loss of a spouse as the most stressful of any life event. Individuals experiencing such a loss must not only cope with loneliness, grief, and financial and legal problems, they must also carve out new social roles and identities as single persons and forge new life styles by themselves.

In her well-known study of widowhood in Chicago, Lopata (1970, 1973, 1975) identified what she called a "society of widows," widows who naturally bonded together to combat loneliness and provide mutual emotional support. More recently, social workers, nurses, and other helping professionals have set up formal programs of support and mutual help groups for widows. In

1970, Phyllis Silverman, a trained social worker, established the Widow-to-Widow Program. The program is guided by the conviction that the best providers of help and support for widows are other widows and is based on the principle of peer support. A widow who has successfully managed her own grief contacts a newly bereaved widow and offers information, advice, and emotional support. Silverman, MacKenzie, Pettipas, and Wilson (1974) have reported favorable results for counselors and counselees alike. The caregiver serves as a role model for the widow and offers a shoulder to cry on and a listening ear. Helpers aid the newly widowed in decision making and problem solving, in coping with loneliness, and in establishing a new life as an independent, functioning individual. The Widow-to-Widow Program, like other effective support groups, offers the widow the opportunity to later function as a helper herself, thus gaining the benefits of providing care for another in need.

Hiltz (1977) started a similar program for widows in July 1970. The Widow Consultation Center in Manhattan offered widows individual counseling and support groups, as well as financial and legal counseling. Weekly discussion groups proved successful in alleviating feelings of loneliness and providing assurance that the widow was not unique, that others had similar problems. Members of the groups cited emotional support as the major benefit obtained from participation. Someone to listen and give sympathy were the benefits most valued by the widows.

Burnside (1978) has described her success with groups of grievers, claiming that such groups help the members by facilitating adjustment to the loss of a spouse and preventing subsequent problems. Kitzinger (1980) similarly has reported success with support groups for individuals who have lost spouses. As a result of their participation in regular group meetings, the members began to deal more realistically with feelings, talked more openly of their depression, and made good friends whom they also saw outside the group. They learned to cope effectively with loneliness through meeting new friends, by discovering new activities, or by learning to be comfortable as a single person.

Reporting on a study of the effectiveness of different types of groups for widows, Barrett (1978) notes that three types of groups are effective: (1) self-help groups (problem focused), (2) confidant groups (focused on building friendships and intimate relations), and (3) consciousness-raising groups (focused on the roles of women in society). Pretests and posttests on a variety of physical and mental health measures were administered to the group members. Analysis of the data revealed positive changes on almost all measures. The reported changes included reduced feelings of unique experience, increased self-confidence, a better future outlook, increased social contacts, and improved physical health. Those in the consciousness-raising groups showed the most significant positive change.

Problems of the Aging Process

In 1959, Stein, a psychiatrist, organized groups of elderly persons who felt lonely and isolated and desired more social life. The groups focused on arranging recreational activities, on helping with family, medical, and economic problems, and on social participation. The groups of five to seven older patients, led by a caseworker, met once a week in a hospital setting. The members focused on practical problems; however, such topics as illness, loneliness, family difficulties, and fear of death were also discussed. After their participation, the members showed improved social participation and social integration (Goldfarb, 1972).

Somewhat later, Burnside (1970a) reported favorable adjustment to major problems of aging through group work. She worked for 18 months with nursing home patients. Her groups focused on loss as a major theme: loss of spouse, physical losses, loss of money, and death, the ultimate loss that all members faced. Based on her group work experience, she concluded that "group work for the aged is indeed useful; it allows patients to discuss and share their losses" (p. 25).

Capuzzi and Fillion (1979) found group counseling with the elderly to be an effective way to increase awareness of the needs of self and others, to accept the aging process as a natural consequence of living rather than as a tragedy, to provide and share information about aging and community resources, to increase positive attitudes toward aging, and to provide emotional support in times of need. Their eight weekly group sessions included various topics for discussion, for example, dealing with loss and loneliness, becoming aware of community resources, finding support from others, and dealing with death. Based on their work, the authors concluded:

> It is our opinion that counseling groups for the elderly could provide an important dimension in the lives of many people who are living alone and facing the aging process without support and understanding from others. These people are faced with loss and loneliness, physical limitations, frustration over their lack of stamina, concern over the possibility of loss of control of their lives, and a sense of urgency about living life to the fullest. All of these concerns could be discussed in group counseling that would allow group members to understand that they are not alone in their needs.

By helping members understand that they are experiencing normal "aging pains" and providing a climate for group support, group members could be aided in adjusting to their positions in life. (p. 154)

Campbell and Chenoweth (1980) experienced similar positive results using a slightly different format. They organized workshops for the elderly that included guest lectures by experts on a topic, followed by group discussion. Peer counselors were also present and worked informally in the workshop groups. Nineteen workshops on sleep, memory, arthritis, nutrition, and other topics of interest to the elderly were conducted. Small support groups grew out of the workshop presentations. For example, a group for people with memory loss was formed following the workshop on that topic. When surveyed after involvement in the program, the participants reported increased knowledge and greater social involvement; and the peer counselors reported greater empathy, better understanding of their own problems, and a sense of achieving something worthwhile.

Opportunities for Growth

Another type of group that provides a valuable experience and opportunities for continued self-exploration by the elderly is the growth group. Senior Actualization and Growth Explorations (SAGE) is a group developed by professionals who wanted to create a growth setting for the elderly. Borrowing from a variety of sources—group therapy, relaxation techniques—SAGE provided an intensive experience involving weekly, three-to-four-hour sessions for nine months for 60 people aged 60 and over. The group offered physical, spiritual, intrapersonal, and interpersonal activities in a climate of strong support. Subsequently, the participants were interviewed to determine the results of the group experience. Pretest and posttest scores from a variety of mental and physical health measures were analyzed to assess change. In their report, Lieberman and Gourash (1979) pointed out that, compared to controls, the participants had greater life satisfaction and self-esteem and lower depression, anxiety, and other psychiatric symptoms. Waters, White, Dates, Reitzer, and Weaver (1979) reported similar positive outcomes from their work on the Oakland Project, which provided growth groups for the well elderly. After participation in the groups, the members changed positively on three attitudes and one behavior—on self-esteem, attitudes about relationship with family, and attitudes about relationships to persons outside the family and on behavior toward persons outside the family.

PRINCIPLES OF EFFECTIVE GROUP WORK

To conduct effective group work with the elderly, several factors must be considered. First, a decision must be made on the nature and purpose of the group—psychoanalytic, social, discussion, humanistic, peer support, theme-specific, growth, activity, reminiscence, or some combination of these. The next important consideration is how to form the group. The type of group will of course dictate to a certain extent how it is to be formed and who will profit from participation. Relevant factors might include group size, sex distribution of the members, their functional capabilities, and their level of psychopathology.

It has been suggested (Dinkmeyer & Moro, 1971) that 16 is the maximum number for a group; the most effective group is probably one of 8 to 10 members. Some groups might achieve the best results if all members are of the same sex; whereas, in other groups, mixed sexes might produce better results. Goldstein (1971) claims that member composition and balance are key variables in the success of a group. In any event, it is important not to include "dangerous" members or members who are so cognitively or physically impaired that they do not really "fit" with other members. For most practitioners dealing with the well elderly in community settings this is not a major problem.

After deciding on composition, it is important to consider time frames, physical setting, leadership, and format of the group. The group should be held at times when the elderly function best, which is usually during the daytime. Evening sessions will not be very successful. The physical setting is also important; the elderly tire more easily and also may have various impairments in eyesight, hearing, and mobility. Uneven temperatures, glare, noise, and uncomfortable furniture should be avoided. The group should be held in a safe location. Access is an important issue, and transportation may have to be provided. Finally, provision should be made for wheelchairs and for those who have difficulty walking.

Leadership is an important variable in group work with the elderly. The leaders need to be very enthusiastic and active to be effective. They should also have some knowledge of aging and be aware of the myths and stereotypes regarding aging and the elderly. The leaders could be chosen from the ranks of those in the group; this is the peer leader concept. Or educated professionals could lead the group. Two leaders might prove more effective than one. Whatever the choice, particular kinds of leadership skills are needed: management skills (structuring a discussion, setting limits on discussion and behavior), caring skills (promoting a positive emotional climate, relieving tension, stressing acceptance, being cooperative, and providing warmth), and meaning attribution skills (giving and interpreting information).

In 1967, Lowy established Recovery, a type of peer support group for released mental patients. Based on his experience with the group, Lowy (1967) cited three important factors in effective group work: authority, structure, and language. The group must have a clear sense of goals and purposes, and there must be some clear-cut form of leadership. The members must speak a common language and share common symbols and meanings. The group's structure must provide a basis for relating and accomplishing group goals. A certain format or standard procedure and use of a common language will serve to provide such a structure.

Based on his experience with groups, Forman (1967) suggests that:

> conflict, controversy, and confrontation applied differentially are useful techniques in working with older adults. Healthy and productive conflict has an invigorating and stimulating effect on older people and can expedite group movement. Dealing with and resolving conflict creates satisfaction, a sense of achievement, and the reality of participating more fully in life. Each successfully resolved conflict increases the group's ability to deal with future conflicts. The behavior of individuals leads one to believe that group successes in this area are internalized by the members. (p. 84)

Groups generally go through several stages of development: orientation, conflict, conflict resolution and harmony, and cohesiveness. This process is sometimes referred to as forming, storming, norming, and conforming. In adapting themselves to these stages, the group members must come to understand and accept each other before any real issue resolution, problem solving, or personal growth and development can take place. The members also need to be prepared for the ending of the group and for resuming life on their own. It is particularly important to come to closure on outstanding issues and tasks before ending the group.

Yalom and Terrazas (1968) and Burnside (1970b, 1978) offer illustrative case examples and concrete suggestions on how to establish groups and conduct group work successfully with the elderly. One particular technique that is very effective is that of peer support or peer counseling (Alpaugh & Haney, 1978; Becker & Zarit, 1978; Bolton & Dignum-Scott, 1979; Salmon, 1979; Silverman, 1970; Waters et al., 1979). Many elderly who reject help offered by a psychologist, psychiatrist, or other professional will accept help from a peer—someone who has been through the same experience or who has the same problem. The use of peer counselors can result in trust and acceptance and also reduce the stigma associated with receiving help from a professional. Also, the generation gap problem is reduced when peer counselors are used. In short, the peer can be an effective model for the elderly person with a problem (M. Romaniuk, Priddy, J. C. Romaniuk, 1981). Thus, female peer counselors have proven remarkably effective with widows. Having experienced widowhood herself, such a counselor understands the needs, problems, and feelings of the widow and can empathize and she can draw upon her own experience to provide practical advice and suggestions.

The peer counselor benefits almost as much from helping as the individual benefits from being helped. Helping another provides an opportunity to express emotion, gain satisfaction, learn better how to deal with people and problems, and gain in understanding, insight, and empathy. In this context, Babic (1972) and others have stressed the need for older individuals to have a choice of roles with the opportunity to change and grow as skill and confidence develop.

M. Romaniuk and Priddy (1980) have successfully trained peer counselors to help widows. Similarly, Silverman et al. (1974) have effectively trained peer counselors for the Widow-to-Widow Program. They cite the following prerequisites for effective peer counseling. The peer counselors must:

- have recovered from their own grief
- be able to talk about it
- have listening skills
- have the "guts" to go out and make the first visit on own initiative
- be secure enough so that they do not feel rejected if the bereaved widow says no or refuses to open the door
- have a commitment to helping others

Schwartz (1980) lists the following additional personal characteristics as essential for peer counselors: being a good listener, exhibiting accurate empathy, and displaying unconditional warmth and genuineness. He has effectively trained individuals to develop such characteristics.

CONCLUSIONS

From our discussion, it is clear that group therapy is an effective instrument for dealing with the many needs and problems of the elderly. Groups are a social phenomenon. Socialization of the individual is continuous throughout all stages of life. But it is never so important as it is when one reaches old age. At that stage, individuals experience biological, psychological, and sociological dysfunctions, although to a varying extent. The elderly must be socialized to new life styles that are often at lower economic levels and to a new world that is everchanging. They may have to adjust to the loss of a spouse, friends, or relatives. Group therapy is a means of helping such individuals adapt to their changed situations. It provides a structure in which they can share experiences with other individuals with similar problems. It allows for feedback, a basic human need. Finally, participation in a group often results in a reciprocal relationship of helping and being helped. It is perhaps this unifying component, more than any other, that makes group therapy a viable social adaptation mechanism for the elderly.

An important objective in the development and use of groups in providing human services for the well elderly is to maintain or reestablish social relationships as they outlive their mates or peers or find it necessary to move to new communities. Other objectives are to provide continued intellectual and social growth, to prevent obsolescence in a rapidly changing world, and to enhance and enrich the elderly's interests and abilities. Most importantly, such groups can provide support through times of crisis, such as a prolonged illness, the loss of some physical capacity, or the prospect of therapy in the family (Hartford, 1980). The need for relationships and social contacts and a sense of belonging and self-perception that spring from normal life support groups may disappear with the loss of a spouse, the death of friends and relatives, or movement away from one's usual social contacts due to hospitalization or institutionalization (Hartford, 1971). In such situations, group participation can help to foster growth in self-awareness, to explore feelings of loss, and ultimately to bring such feelings to the surface in order to deal with grief. Group therapy helps the participants see themselves through others via common feelings and emotions, and the circumstances that are commonplace among the nation's elderly.

Finally, the group method can provide an enhanced, improved, or restored sense of self and identity through positive feedback from other group members. It thus can provide collective support through crises and trauma, induction to new roles or substitute roles, the establishment of new relationships, and the creation of opportunities for new social affiliations and new friends (Hartford, 1980).

For the interested reader, Appendixes 7–A and 7–B contain a list of selected support groups currently providing aid to the afflicted elderly in the various areas discussed in this chapter.

REFERENCES

Alpaugh, P., & Haney, M. (1978). *Counseling the older adult—A training manual*. Los Angeles: University of Southern California, Andrus Center.

Atchley, R. C. (1976). *The sociology of retirement*. New York: John Wiley & Sons.

Babic, A. (1972). The older volunteer: Expectations and satisfactions. *Gerontologist, 12,* 87–93.

Barrett, C. J. (1978). Effectiveness of widows' groups in facilitating change. *Journal of Counseling and Clinical Psychology, 46,* 20–31.

Barton, M. G. (1962). Group counseling with older hospital patients. *Gerontologist, 2,* 51–56.

Beaulieu, E. M., & Karpinski, J. (1981). Group treatment of elderly with ill spouses. *Social Casework, 63,* 551–557.

Becker, F., & Zarit, S. (1978). Training older adults as peer counselors. *Educational Gerontology, 3,* 241–250.

Bednar, R., & Kaul, T. (1978). Experimental group research: Current perspectives. In S. Garfield & A. Bergin (Eds.), *Handbook of psychotherapy and behavior change* (2nd ed), pp. 769–815. New York: John Wiley & Sons.

Benaim, S. (1957). Group psychotherapy within a geriatric unit: An experiment. *International Journal of Social Psychiatry, 3,* 123–128.

Bolton, C., & Dignum-Scott, J. (1979). Peer group advocacy counseling for the elderly. *Journal of Gerontological Social Work, 1*(4), 321–331.

Burnside, I. M. (1969). Group work among the aged. *Nursing Outlook, 9,* 68–71.

Burnside, I. M. (1970a). Loss: A constant theme in group work with the aged. *Hospital and Community Psychiatry, 21*(6), 173–177.

Burnside, I. M. (1970b). Group work with the aged: Selected literature. *Gerontologist, 10,* 241–246.

Burnside, I. M. (1971). Long-term group work with the hospitalized aged. *Gerontologist, 11,* 213–218.

Burnside, I. M. (1978). *Working with the elderly: Group processes and techniques.* North Scituate, Mass.: Duxubury Press.

Campbell, R., & Chenoweth, B. (1980, November). *Peer support system.* Paper presented at the 33rd annual scientific meeting of the Gerontological Society of America, San Diego, Calif.

Caplan, G. (1974) *A study of natural support systems.* Unpublished manuscript, Harvard Medical School, Laboratory of Community Psychiatry, Boston, Mass.

Caplan, G. (1976). The family as a support system. In G. Caplan & M. Killilea (Eds.), *Support systems and mutual help: Multidisciplinary explorations* (pp. 19–36). New York: Grune & Stratton.

Caplan, G., & Killilea, M. (Eds.). (1976). *Support systems and mutual help: Multidisciplinary explorations.* New York: Grune & Stratton.

Capuzzi, D., & Fillion, N. (1979). Group counseling for the elderly. *Journal for Specialists in Group Work, 4,* 148–154.

Capuzzi, D., & Gross, D. (1980). Group work with the elderly: An overview for counselors. *Personnel and Guidance Journal,* 206–211.

Cassel, J. C. (1974). Psychiatric epidemiology. In G. Caplan (Ed.), *American handbook of psychiatry* (Vol. 2, pp. 401–411). New York: Basic Books.

Dinkmeyer, D. C., & Moro, J.J. (1971). *Group counseling: Theory and practice.* Itasca, Ill.: F. E. Peacock.

Eisdorfer, C., & Stotsky, B. A. (1977). Intervention, treatment and rehabilitation of psychiatric disorders. In J. E. Birren & K. W. Schaie (Eds.), *Handbook of the psychology of aging* (pp. 724–740). New York: Van Nostrand Reinhold.

Forman, M. (1967). Conflict, controversy, and confrontation in group work with older adults. *Social Work, 12,* 84.

Frank, J. D. (1973). *Persuasion and healing: A comparative study of psychotherapy* (rev. ed.). Baltimore, Md.: Johns Hopkins University Press.

Franzino, M. A., Geren, J. J., & Meiman, G. L. (1976). Group discussion among the terminally ill. *International Journal of Group Psychotherapy, 26*(1), 43–48.

Goldfarb, A. (1972). Group therapy with the old and aged. In H. I. Kaplan & B. J. Sadock (Eds.), *Group treatment of mental illness* (pp. 113–131). New York: Dalton.

Goldstein, A. P. (1971). *Psychotherapeutic attraction.* New York: Pergamon Press.

Hartford, M. E. (1971). *Groups in social work: Applications of small group research to social work practice.* New York: Columbia University Press.

Hartford, M. E. (1980). The use of group methods for work with the aged. In J. E. Birren & R. Sloane (Eds.), *Handbook of mental health and aging* (pp. 806–826). Englewood Cliffs, N.J.: Prentice-Hall.

Havighurst, R. J. (1961). The nature and values of meaningful free-time activity. In R. W. Kleemeier (Ed.), *Aging and leisure* (pp. 309–344). New York: Oxford University Press.

Hendricks, J., & Hendricks, C. D. (1977). *Aging in mass society: Myths and realities.* Cambridge, Mass.: Winthrop.

Hiltz, S. R. (1977). *Creating community services for widows.* Port Washington, N.Y.: Rennikat Press.

Holmes, T., & Rahe, R. H. (1967). The social readjustment scale. *Journal of Psychosomatic Research, 2,* 213–217.

Horton, A. M., & Linden, M. E. (1982). Geriatric group psychotherapy. In A. Horton (Ed.), *Mental health interventions for the aging* (pp. 51–68). New York: Praeger Press.

Kahn, R. L., & Antonucci, T. C. (1979). *Convoys over the life course: Attachments, roles, and social support.* Ann Arbor: University of Michigan, Institute for Social Research.

Kaplan, J. (1953). *A social program for older people.* Minneapolis, Minn.: Lund Press.

Kastenbaum, R. (1964). The reluctant therapist. In R. Kastenbaum (Ed.), *New thoughts on old age* (pp. 139–145). New York: Springer.

Kastenbaum, R. (1966). The mental life of dying geriatric patients. *Proceedings of the seventh international conference on gerontology* (pp. 153–159).

Katz, M. (1972). Self-help groups. *Social Work, 17*(6), 120–121.

Kaul, T., & Bednar, R. (1978). Conceptualizing group research: A preliminary analysis. *Small Group Behavior, 9,* 173–191.

Knight, B. (1979). Psychotherapy and behavior change with the noninstitutionalized aged. *International Journal of Aging and Human Development, 9,* 221–236.

Kramer, M., Taube, A., & Redick, R W. (1973). Patterns of use of psychiatric facilities by the aged: Past, present, and future. In C. Eisdorfer & M. Lawton (Eds.), *The psychology of adult development and aging* (pp. 428–528). Washington, D.C.: American Psychological Association.

Kropotkin, P. (1925). *Mutual aid.* Boston, Mass.: Extending Horizon Books. (Original work published 1914)

Kubie, S., & Landau, G. (1953). *Group work with the aged.* New York: International Universities Press.

Lenneberg, E., & Rowbotham, J. L. (1970). *The ileostomy patient.* Springfield, Ill.: Charles C Thomas.

Lieberman, M. A., & Gourash, N. (1979). Evaluating the effects of change on the elderly. *International Journal of Group Psychotherapy, 29,* 283–304.

Lieberman, M. A., Yalom, I. D., & Miles, M. B. (1973). *Encounter groups: First facts.* New York: Basic Books.

Linden, M. E. (1956). The older person in the family. *Social Casework, 37,* 75–81.

Lopata, H. Z. (1970). The social involvement of American widows. *American Behavioral Scientist, 14,* 41–57.

Lopata, H. Z. (1973). *Widowhood in an American city.* Cambridge, Mass.: Schenkman.

Lopata, H. Z. (1975). Support systems of elderly urbanites: Chicago of the 1970's. *Gerontologist, 15,* 35–41.

Lowenthal, M. F., & Robinson, B. (1976). Social networks and isolation. In R. H. Binstock & E. Shanas (Eds.), *Handbook of aging and the social sciences* (pp. 432–456). New York: Van Nostrand Reinhold.

Lowy, L. (1967). Roadblocks in group work practice with older people: A framework for analysis. *Gerontologist, 2,* 109–113.

Lucas, C. (1964). Group leadership. In C. Lucas (Ed.), *Recreation in gerontology* (pp. 14–24). Springfield, Ill.: Charles C. Thomas.

Mardoyan, J. L., & Weiss, D. M. (1981). The efficacy of group counseling with older adults. *Personnel and Guidance Journal, 60,* 161–163.

Mizruchi, E. H. (1964). *Success and opportunity.* New York: Free Press.

National Association of Social Workers. (1980). *Social group work with older people.* New York: Arno Press. (original work published 1961)

Petty, B. J., Moeller, T. P., & Campbell, R. Z. (1976). Support groups for elderly persons in the community. *Gerontologist, 16*(6), 522–528.

Pilsuk, M., & Minkler, M. (1980). Supportive networks: Life ties for the elderly. *Journal of Social Issues, 36*(2), 95–116.

Pomeroy, E. L. (1972). Group psychotherapy in old age: Chance for creative intervention. *Geriatric Focus.*

Pratt, J. H. (1907). The class method of treating consumption in the homes of the poor. *Journal of the American Medical Association, 49,* 755–757.

Romaniuk, M., & Priddy, J. M. (1980). Widowhood peer counseling. *Counseling and Values, 24*(3), 195–203.

Romaniuk, M., Priddy, J. M., & Romaniuk, J. C. (1981). Older peer counselor training. *Counselor Education and Supervision, 26,* 225–231.

Ronch, J. L., & Maizler, I. S. (1977). Individual psychotherapy with the institutionalized aged. *American Journal of Orthopsychiatry, 47,* 275–283.

Rosin, A. J. (1975). Group discussion: A therapeutic tool in a chronic disease hospital. *Geriatrics, 30,* 45–48.

Rosow I. (1967). Social integration of the aged. New York: Free Press.

Ross, M. (1975). Community geriatric group therapies: A comprehensive review. In M. Rosenbaum & M. M. Berger (Eds.), *Group psychotherapy and group function* (pp. 500–520). New York: Basic Books.

Salmon, R. (1979). The older volunteer. *Journal of Gerontological Social Work, 2*(1), 67–75.

Saul, S. R., & Saul, S. (1974). Group psychotherapy in a proprietary nursing home. *Gerontologist, 14,* 446–450.

Scheidlinger, S. (1968). Therapeutic group approaches in community mental health. *Social Work, 13*(2), 87–95.

Schwartz, A. (1980). Training of peer counselors. In S. S. Sargent (Ed.), *Nontraditional therapy and counseling with the aging* (pp. 146–160). New York: Springer.

Schwartz, E. D., & Goodman, J. I. (1952). Group therapy of obesity in elderly diabetics. *Geriatrics, 7*, 280–283.

Shore, H. (1964). Group work and recreation. In G. Gazda (Ed.), *Innovations to group psychotherapy.* New York: Putnam & Sons.

Silver, A. (1950). Group psychotherapy with senile psychotic patients. *Geriatrics, 5*, 147–150.

Silverman, P. S. (1970). The widow as a caregiver in a program of preventive intervention with other widows. *Mental Hygiene, 54*, 540–547.

Silverman, P. S., & Cooperband, A. (1975). On widowhood mutual help and the elderly widow. *Journal of Geriatric Psychiatry, 8*(1), 9–27.

Silverman, P. S., MacKenzie, D., Pettipas, M., & Wilson, E. (Eds.). (1974). *Helping each other in widowhood.* New York: Miller Press.

Stein, A. (1959, January). *Group psychotherapy in a general hospital: Principles and practice.* Paper presented at the annual meeting of the American Group Psychotherapy Association, New York, N. Y.

Stichman, J. A., & Schoenberg, J. (1972). Heart wife counselors. *Omega, 3*(3), 155–161.

Sussman, M. (1976). The family life of old people. In R. H. Binstock & E. Shanas (Eds.), *Handbook of aging and the social sciences* (pp. 218–243). New York: Van Nostrand Reinhold.

Traunstein, D. M., & Steinman, R. (1973). Voluntary self-help organizations: An exploratory study. *Journal of Voluntary Action Research, 2*(4), 230–239.

Verwoerdt, A. (1976). *Clinical geropsychiatry.* Baltimore, Md.: Williams & Wilkins.

Vickers, G. (1971). Institutional and personal roles. *Human Relations, 24*(5), 433–447.

Waters, E., White, B., Dates, B., Reitzer, S., & Weaver, A. (1979). *Peer group counseling for older people.* Rochester, Mich.: Oakland University Continuum Center.

Weiss, R S. (1976). Transition states and other stressful situations: Their nature and programs for their management. In G. Caplan & M. Killilea (Eds.), *Support systems and mutual help: Multidisciplinary explorations* (pp. 213–222). New York: Grune & Stratton.

Wolff, K. (1957). Group psychotherapy with geriatric patients in a mental hospital. *Journal of the American Geriatrics Society, 5*, 13–19.

Wolff, K. (1963). Individual psychotherapy with geriatric patients. *Diseases of the Nervous System, 24*, 688–691.

Yalom, I. D. (1970). *The theory and practice of group psychotherapy.* New York: Basic Books.

Yalom, I. D., & Terrazas, F. (1968). Group therapy for psychotic elderly patients. *American Journal of Nursing, 68*, 1690–1694.

Zarit, S. (1980). Group and family intervention. In S. Zarit (Ed.), *Aging and mental disorders* (pp. 322–350). New York: Free Press.

Appendix 7-A

National Offices of Support Groups

Alzheimer's Disease and Related
  Disorders Association
National Headquarters
360 North Michigan Avenue
Chicago, Illinois 60601
1-800-621-1379

American Cancer Society
National Headquarters
777 Third Avenue
New York, New York 10017
1-800-552-7996

The Mended Hearts, Inc.
7320 Greenville Avenue
Dallas, Texas 75231
(214) 750-5442

Widowed Persons Service
c/o American Association of Retired Persons
1909 K Street, N.W.
Suite 584
Washington, D.C. 20049
(202) 872-4700

Appendix 7-B

State Divisions of the American Cancer Society

Alabama Division, Inc.
2926 Central Avenue
Birmingham, Alabama 35209
(205) 879-2242

Alaska Division, Inc.
1343 G Street
Anchorage, Alaska 99501
(907) 277-8696

Arizona Division, Inc.
634 West Indian School Road
P.O. Box 33187
Phoenix, Arizona 85067
(602) 264-5861

Arkansas Division, Inc.
5520 West Markham Street
P.O. Box 3822
Little Rock, Arkansas 72203
(501) 664-3480-1-2

California Division, Inc.
1710 Webster Street
P.O. Box 2061
Oakland, California 94604
(415) 893-7900

Colorado Division, Inc.
1809 East 18th Avenue
P.O. Box 18268
Denver, Colorado 80218
(303) 321-2464

Connecticut Division, Inc.
Barnes Park South
14 Village Lane
P.O. Box 410
Wallingford, Connecticut 06492
(203) 265-7161

Delaware Division, Inc.
1708 Lovering Avenue
Suite 202
Wilmington, Delaware 19806
(302) 654-6267

District of Columbia Division, Inc.
Universal Building, South
1825 Connecticut Avenue, N.W.
Washington, D.C. 20009
(202) 483-2600

Florida Division, Inc.
1001 South MacDill Avenue
Tampa, Florida 33609
(813) 253-0541

Georgia Division, Inc.
1422 W. Peachtree Street, N.W.
Atlanta, Georgia 30309
(404) 892-0076

Hawaii Division, Inc.
Community Services Center Bldg.
200 North Vineyard Boulevard
Honolulu, Hawaii 96817
(808) 531-1662-3-4-5

Idaho Division, Inc.
1609 Abbs Street
P.O. Box 5386
Boise, Idaho 83705
(208) 343-4609

Illinois Division, Inc.
37 South Wabash Avenue
Chicago, Illinois 60603
(312) 372-0472

Indiana Division, Inc.
4755 Kingsway Drive, Suite 100
Indianapolis, Indiana 46205
(317) 257-5326

Iowa Division, Inc.
Highway #18 West
P.O. Box 980
Mason City, Iowa 50401
(515) 423-0712

Kansas Division, Inc.
3003 Van Buren Street
Topeka, Kansas 66611
(913) 267-0131

Kentucky Division, Inc.
Medical Arts Bldg.
1169 Eastern Parkway
Louisville, Kentucky 40217
(502) 459-1867

Louisiana Division, Inc.
Masonic Temple Bldg., Room 810
333 St. Charles Avenue
New Orleans, Louisiana 70130
(504) 523-2029

Maine Division, Inc.
52 Federal Street
Brunswick, Maine 04011
(207) 729-3339

Maryland Division, Inc.
1840 York Road
Timonium, Maryland 21093
(301) 561-4790

Massachusetts Division, Inc.
247 Commonwealth Avenue
Boston, Massachusetts 02116
(617) 267-2650

Mississippi Division, Inc.
345 North Mart Plaza
Jackson, Mississippi 39206
(601) 362-8874

Michigan Division, Inc.
1205 East Saginaw Street
Lansing, Michigan 48906
(507) 371-2920

Minnesota Division, Inc.
3316 West 66th Street
Minneapolis, Minnesota 55435
(612) 925-2772

Missouri Division, Inc.
3322 American Avenue
P.O. Box 1066
Jefferson City, Missouri 65102
(314) 893-4800

Montana Division, Inc.
2820 First Avenue South
Billings, Montana 59101
(406) 252-7111

Nebraska Division, Inc.
8502 West Center Road
Omaha, Nebraska 68124
(402) 393-5800

Nevada Division, Inc.
1325 E. Harmon Avenue
Las Vegas, Nevada 89109
(702) 798-6877

New Hampshire Division, Inc.
686 Mast Road
Manchester, New Hampshire 03102
(603) 669-3270

New Jersey Division, Inc.
2600 Route 1
CN2201
North Brunswick, New Jersey 08902
(201) 297-8000

New Mexico Division, Inc.
5800 Lomas Blvd., N.E.
Albuquerque, New Mexico 87110
(505) 262-2336

New York State Division, Inc.
6725 Lyons Street
P.O. Box 7
East Syracuse, New York 13057
(315) 437-7025

Long Island Division, Inc.
535 Broad Hollow Road
(Route 110)
Melville, New York 11747
(516) 420-1111

New York City Division, Inc.
19 West 56th Street
New York, New York 10019
(212) 586-8700

Queens Division, Inc.
111-15 Queens Boulevard
Forest Hills, New York 11375
(718) 263-2224

Westchester Division, Inc.
901 North Broadway
White Plains, New York 10603
(914) 949-4800

North Carolina Division, Inc.
222 North Person Street
P.O. Box 27624
Raleigh, North Carolina 27611
(919) 834-8463

North Dakota Division, Inc.
Hotel Graver Annex Bldg.
115 Roberts Street
P.O. Box 426
Fargo, North Dakota 58102
(701) 232-1385

Ohio Division, Inc.
1375 Euclid Avenue
Suite 312
Cleveland, Ohio 44115
(216) 771-6700

Oklahoma Division, Inc.
3800 N. Cromley
Oklahoma City, Oklahoma 73112
(405) 946-5000

Oregon Division, Inc.
0330 S. W. Curry
Portland, Oregon 97201
(503) 295-6422

Pennsylvania Division, Inc.
Route 422 & Sipe Avenue
P.O. Box 416
Hershey, Pennsylvania 17033
(717) 533-6144

Philadelphia Division, Inc.
21 South 12th Street
Philadelphia, Pennsylvania 19107
(215) 665-2900

Puerto Rico Division, Inc.
(Avenue Domenech 273
Halo Rey, P.R.)
GPO Box 6004
San Juan, Puerto Rico 00936
(809) 764-2295

Rhode Island Division, Inc.
345 Blackstone Blvd.
Providence, Rhode Island 02900
(401) 831-6970

South Carolina Division, Inc.
2442 Devine Street
Columbia, South Carolina 29205
(803) 256-0245

South Dakota Division, Inc.
1025 North Minnesota Avenue
Hillcrest Plaza
Sioux Falls, South Dakota 57104
(605) 336-0897

Tennessee Division, Inc.
713 Melpark Drive
Nashville, Tennessee 37204
(615) 383-1710

Texas Division, Inc.
3834 Spicewood Springs Road
P.O. Box 9863
Austin, Texas 78766
(512) 345-4560

Utah Division, Inc.
610 East South Temple
Salt Lake City, Utah 84012
(801) 322-0431

Vermont Division, Inc.
13 Loomis Street, Drawer C
Montpelier, Vermont 05602
(802) 223-2348

Virginia Division, Inc.
3218 West Cary Street
P.O. Box 7288
Richmond, Virginia 23221
(804) 359-0208

Washington Division, Inc.
2120 First Avenue North
Seattle, Washington 98109
(206) 283-1152

West Virginia Division, Inc.
Suite 100
240 Capital Street
Charleston, West Virginia 25301
(301) 344-3611

Wisconsin Division, Inc.
615 North Sherman Avenue
P.O. Box 8370
Madison, Wisconsin 53708
(608) 249-0487

Milwaukee Division, Inc.
6401 West Capitol Drive
Milwaukee, Wisconsin 53216
(414) 461-1100

Wyoming Division, Inc.
Indian Hills Center
506 Shoshoni
Cheyenne, Wyoming 82009
(307) 638-3331

Chapter 8

Reminiscence and Life Review Therapy

> They live by memory rather than hope, for what is left to them of life is but little compared to the long past. This again is the cause of their loquacity. They are continually talking of the past, because they enjoy remembering.

> Aristotle, *Rhetoric.*

As Butler (1963b) points out, our culture devalues memories or recollections of the old. We condemn the old for living in the past, entering a second childhood, or denying reality if they choose to reminisce and talk of past life events, experiences, people, and places. We even pejoratively and incorrectly tend to link active reminiscing with loneliness, tenacious and inappropriate clinging to a previous identity, or senility (Lewis & Butler, 1974).

Yet our artistic and philosophical tradition places a higher value on memory and reminiscence (Butler, 1963b). Literature is replete with beautiful examples of reminiscence and life review. Hemingway's *The Snows of Kilimanjaro* and Tolstoy's *The Death of Ivan Ilych* are two of the best examples. Indeed, published reminiscences by such famous people as Benjamin Franklin, Henry Adam, and Igor Stravinsky have been well received by the public.

In his novel *Ada*, Vladimir Nabokov makes a very positive statement on the value of memory and remembering: "Time is but memory in the making. To be means to know one has been" (Butler, 1971, p. 49–50). Goethe similarly noted the values of reflecting on the past: "He is the happiest man who can see the connection between the end and the beginning of his life" (Butler, 1963, p. 523). This positive view of the uses of the past underlies the therapeutic role of reminiscence and the life review as effective intervention techniques with the elderly. In this chapter, we review the relevant empirical literature on reminiscence and life review therapy, particularly those studies related to depression, self-concept, self-esteem, and the morale of the elderly. In this context, we offer some practical guidelines on how to conduct life review therapy with the elderly.

THEORETICAL PERSPECTIVES

Reminiscence may be defined as "the act, process, or fact of recalling or remembering the past" (Butler, 1964, p. 266). When reminiscing, one is remembering past life events, experiences, people, and places. The activity can be mental or verbal. One may recall thoughts or feelings, even smells or sounds, connected with the past. Thoughts of the past may emerge as "stray, seemingly insignificant thoughts about self or may become continuous" (Butler, 1971, p. 49). Reminiscence may produce nostalgia, pleasure, an idealized past, or mild regret. On the other hand, it may lead to anxiety, guilt, depression, or despair. "Memory pains us and shames us and entertains us and serves the sense of self and its continuity" (Butler, 1964, p. 266).

The term *life review* has gained wide recognition through the writings of Robert Butler, former director of the National Institute on Aging. Life review encompasses reminiscence, but includes much more. It is:

> a naturally occurring, universal mental process characterized by the progressive return to consciousness of past experiences, and, particularly, the resurgence of unresolved conflicts; simultaneously, and normally, these revived experiences and conflicts can be surveyed and reintegrated. Presumably this process is prompted by the realization of approaching dissolution and death, and the inability to maintain one's sense of personal invulnerability. It is further shaped by contemporaneous experiences and its nature and outcome are affected by the lifelong unfolding of character.
>
> The life review, as a looking-back process that has been set in motion by looking forward to death, potentially proceeds toward personality reorganization. Thus, the life review is not synonymous with, but includes reminiscence; it is not alone either the unbidden return of memories, or the purposive seeking of them although both may occur. (Butler, 1964, pp. 487–488)

In a life review one does not just remember the past; one analyzes, evaluates, restructures, and reconstructs past life events and experiences and their meanings in order to arrive at a better understanding of one's life. The process puts the past into coherent order and proper perspective in light of present values, attitudes, and life experiences. The life review—more common in late life but apparent in all life stages—is thus an active process of personality reorganization. Birren (1964) describes it as "setting one's house in order." During life review, the elderly "integrate life as it has been lived in relation to how it might have been lived" (p. 275).

Socrates recognized the importance of life review in his classic statement that "the unexamined life is not worth living" (Dangott & Kalish, 1979, p. 56). Sigmund Freud referred to neurotic illnesses as "diseases of reminiscence" (Butler, 1963a, p. 523) suggesting the therapeutic value of remembering and the psychopathology of repressing, forgetting, or removing memories from conscious awareness. In the same vein, Butler (1963b) noted that "recovering important memories is a basic ingredient of the curative process in psychoanalysis and necessary for change" (p. 525). In this view, reminiscence and life review are a natural form of personal psychotherapy.

Jung (1934) suggested that the life review helps to reduce psychic tension and restore psychic balance and is necessary to personality development. More specifically, Butler (1963b) described it as a necessary and therapeutic process that begins about age 45, the age at which life's goals are either realized or not. At that age, according to Buhler (1959), internal matters become more important, and self-assessment is initiated in order to restore a sense of personal balance and inner order. This process of self-review results in a sense of either personal fulfillment or personal failure.

Influenced by the earlier work of Sigmund Freud and Charlotte Buhler, Erik Erikson (1950) developed his well-known theory of the eight stages of human development—basically a theory of identity and personality development. Erikson posits that at each life stage the individual must successfully resolve the predominant psychological crisis of the ego in order to move successfully to the next stage. He considered identity formation as a lifelong process; during late life, the major crisis is integrity versus despair. "Reminiscence is hypothesized to be the outcome of the fundamental need of the ego to achieve integrity over despair" (Bielby & Boden, 1981, p. 2). In order to achieve integrity, older individuals must review their lives and determine whether they were inevitable, meaningful, and worthy. If they accept their lives and feel they have done all they could and do not wish anything different, they will achieve integrity over despair and gain wisdom.

Butler and his followers, particularly Myrna Lewis, have done much to make physicians and other practitioners aware of the therapeutic value of reminiscence and life review, and to lay the groundwork for conducting life review therapy with the elderly. Butler (1968) describes the adaptive functions of the life review in the following words:

As the past marches in review, it is surveyed, observed, and reflected upon by the ego. Reconsideration of previous experiences and their meanings occurs, often with concomitant revised or expanded understanding. Such reorganization of past experience may provide a more valid picture, giving new and significant meanings to one's life; it may also prepare one for death, mitigating one's fears.

Although it is not possible at present to describe in detail either the life review or the possibilities for reintegration which are suggested, it seems likely that in the majority of the elderly a substantial reorganization of the personality does occur. This may help to account for the evolution of such qualities as wisdom and serenity, long noted in some of the aged.... In addition to the more impressive constructure aspects of the life review, certain adaptive and defensive aspects may be noted. Some of the aged have illusions of the "good past;" some fantasy the past rather than the future in the service of avoiding the realities of the present; some maintain a characteristic detachment from others and themselves. Although these mechanisms are not constructive, they do assist in maintaining a status quo of psychological functioning (pp. 489–490).

Thus, reminiscence and life review may be therapeutic for the individual. They allow one to address critically and to put in proper perspective such personal issues as the meaning of life and one's existence, past successes and failures in life, past personal problems, and unresolved psychological issues and conflicts, thereby providing new meaning and significance to life. As Lewis & Butler (1974) note, "Reminiscence has a positive function, a psychotherapeutic one, in which the older person reflects on his life in order to resolve, reorganize, and reintegrate what is troubling or preoccupying him" (p. 165).

By reviewing and analyzing past life events, older persons can clearly identify and come to grips with mistakes, wrongdoings, and missed chances and their meanings and thereby gain a revised or expanded understanding of the past (Butler, 1963a). They can express guilt, grief, uncertainty, fear, and uneasiness—tied to their concerns about their effectiveness as parents through the life review (Butler, 1980–1981). When this leads to resolution of past conflicts and psychological issues (which is not always the case), the ego is strengthened and personality reorganization is possible. In addition, the life review results quite naturally in increased self-awareness and self-understanding, the achievement of insight, and the development of creativity, candor, serenity, wisdom, atonement, philosophical development, and maturity (Butler, 1961, 1963b, 1964). Other possible benefits of the life review are a change in character; the righting of old wrongs; reconciliation with enemies; a new sense of candor and honesty that replaces old deceits; and a lively capacity to live in the present, with a renewed sense of awe and wonder and appreciation of nature, beauty, and the arts—a state that may be described as "elementality" (Butler, 1963b). Finally, Butler (1964) suggests that reminiscence and the life review provide a pleasant form of escape, a way to occupy the elderly and fill the voids in their lives. When one is sick and lonely, facing the death of loved ones and the prospect of one's own death, the past can be a comfortable, familiar place to escape to.

Although Butler focuses primarily on the benefits and therapeutic values of reminiscence and the life review, he also describes the negative feelings that can result from it. Such feelings can arise in those who tended to live for the future rather than the present and who are now facing their last years with their hopes still unfulfilled; those who have purposely hurt others and have real guilt; and those who are narcissistic and egoistic and cannot handle death (Butler, 1964). It may be necessary to minimize reminiscence for these individuals because it is too painful.

REVIEW OF EMPIRICAL STUDIES

Despite the benefits of reminiscence and life review cited in the literature, very little empirical research has been conducted to test such claims. The research that has been done (mostly since 1970) has been criticized on several grounds, particularly with respect to limited and small samples and confusion over definitions of the major concepts, reminiscence and life review. In reviewing the following studies, these methodological flaws should be kept in mind.

Based on clinical data collected from a large-scale study of human aging conducted at the National Institute of Mental Health from 1955 to 1961, Butler reported several examples of positive personal change in subjects after they engaged in reminiscence and life review. The therapeutic benefits ranged from a better ability to cope with aging and death to greatly improved relations with family members. Based on his clinical observations, Butler concluded that "people get much out of the opportunity to express thoughts and feelings to someone willing to listen" (Butler, 1980–1981, p. 37).

In an early study on the effects of reminiscence on depression and adjustment, McMahon and Rhudick (1967) noted high correlations between frequency of reminiscence, freedom from depression, and survival one year after the study. They noted:

Reminiscing has an adaptive function and . . . appears to be a complex organized mental activity operating under the control of the ego. . . . It is positively correlated with successful adaptation . . . through maintaining self-esteem, reaffirming a sense of identity, working through and mastering personal losses and contributing positively to society. (p. 28)

McMahon and Rhudick (1967) divided their subjects into groups depending on how they used reminiscence and discovered several uses. The best adjusted subjects used reminiscence for storytelling, which seemed to be a way of relating to others in a meaningful way in the present.

They . . . recount past exploits and experiences with obvious pleasure and in a way which is both entertaining and informative. They seem to have no need to depreciate the present or glorify the past, but they do reminisce actively. The older person's knowledge of a bygone era provides him with the unique opportunity both to preserve his own self-esteem and to contribute to his present society. This group of our subjects seemed best adjusted to senescence with no evidence of depression or excessive denial. (McMahon & Rhudick, 1967, p. 296)

Based on a study of reminiscence among 24 white males aged 65 and over, Lewis (1971) concluded that reminiscence is positively related to maintaining self-concept, especially in times of pervasive stress. He found that reminiscence helps one get through various life crises, particularly the loss of a spouse. Parkes (1970), Lieberman and Falk (1971), and C. H. Kramer, J. Kramer, and Dunlop (1966) identified reminiscence as important in doing necessary grief work and coping with the loss of a loved one. Lewis (1971) argues that consistency of self-concept contributes to positive adaptation and a healthy adjustment to aging "by sustaining an awareness of self and allowing one to recapture valued parts of the self-image" (p. 243). He suggests that "one's memory bank, built over a lifetime of living, is a useful resource in late life for maintaining a sense of worth and interest" (p. 243). Thus, "reminiscence may be ego-supportive by enabling the old person to identify with past accomplishments and to avoid the discrepancy in self-concept that old age represents to a formerly engaged and active member of society" (p. 243). Based on their study of a group of individuals aged 62 and over, Havighurst and Glasser (1972) concluded that there is an association between frequency of reminiscence, positive psychological effects, and personal-social adaptation to aging.

In 1974, Coleman conducted one of the most systematic studies of reminiscence reported in the literature. His sample consisted of 23 men and 25 women between the ages of 62 and 92. Coleman found that those who engaged in a life review were better adjusted than those who did not; this was particularly true of those who were not satisfied with their past lives. Coleman suggests that the life review aids in working through past conflicts. Based on his study, he identified three functions of reminiscence and the life review for elderly subjects: (1) to bring forth a variety of interesting past experiences that could be shared with others or simply enjoyed, (2) to bring some emotional and cognitive clarification to life experiences, and (3) to reveal positive characteristics of the past, thus putting the present in a more favorable light.

Boylin, Gordon, and Nehrke (1976) studied 41 institutionalized veterans to determine the effects of reminiscence on ego adjustment. They administered a questionnaire to the veterans to determine the nature and frequency of reminiscence and a scale to assess ego adjustment. Their study represents a pioneer attempt to define operationally and to measure empirically Erikson's theoretical construct of ego integrity. They found that those who reminisced more frequently scored higher on the measure of ego integrity than those who seldom or never reminisced, thus establishing a link between reminiscence and successful adjustment in late life.

In a recent study, M. Romaniuk and J. Romaniuk (1981) attempted to identify various functions that reminiscence serves for the elderly and also to identify the particular "triggers" that start the process. A factor analysis on data collected from 91 subjects aged 58 to 98 who resided in three retirement communities yielded three factors: Self Regard/Image Enhancement, Present Problem Solving, and Existential Self Understanding. As a reason for engaging in reminiscence, the Self Regard/Image Enhancement factor was acknowledged by the largest number of subjects. Most used reminiscence as a pleasurable form of self-stimulation, a means of bolstering self-worth, a method of self-identification, or a means of entertainment. Significantly fewer used it as a means of solving present problems or dealing with philosophical concerns. The authors concluded that "interpersonal reminiscence appears to be a pleasant activity and is essentially a method of bolstering self-esteem during the course of social interactions. Apparently, self-esteem is maintained through recollections which demonstrate current personal worth and utility or past worth" (p. 68).

The major reminiscence trigger identified by M. Romaniuk and J. Romaniuk (1981) was awareness of death. The next two most frequent triggers were realization of life's goals or accomplishments and the realization of biological decline.

Taken as a whole, the empirical literature suggests that reminiscence and life review are therapeutic and can aid in coping with loss or stress, combating depression, maintaining self-esteem and self-concept, and fostering morale and positive adjustment to aging.

LIFE REVIEW THERAPY

Keen and Fox (1973) have noted that:

> repressed memories . . . won't stay down. To be alive is to have a past. Our only choice is whether we will repress or recreate the past. Childhood may be distant, but it is never quite lost; as full-grown men and women we carry tiny laughing and whimpering children around inside us. We either repress the past and continue to fight its wars with new personnel or we invite it into awareness so that we may see how it has shaped the present. (pp. 41–42)

In the context of this perspective of the important impact of past experiences on current well-being, therapists have been experimenting with the use of life review in individual and group psychotherapy. Life review therapy is defined by Lewis and Butler (1974) as a psychoanalytically oriented action process in which the therapist does not initiate a process but rather "taps into an already ongoing self-analysis and participates in it with the older person" (p. 166). In their view, the major purpose of a psychotherapeutic intervention through life review is "to make it more conscious, deliberate, and efficient" (p. 166). The technique is an effective way to get the elderly to do necessary developmental work of late life, primarily achieving integrity over despair and coming to terms with death. Reedy and Birren (1980) suggest that:

> Life Review . . . is a central developmental task for older adults. Interestingly, the personal consequences of a failure to accomplish this task resemble the characteristics of depression (despair, hopelessness, negative view of self, immobility, feelings of alienation and social isolation). This suggests that providing the opportunity to accomplish the life review may be useful in treating or preventing depression. In this view, occasions for older people to present their life stories need to be systematically and deliberately constructed. (p. 1)

Thus, life review therapy helps the elderly put their pasts into perspective in the light of present events, values, and attitudes. It allows them to experience and acknowledge important emotions and to integrate them into the self, which is essential for healthy functioning. The intervention strategy can be used to help reduce loneliness, enhance self-esteem, increase morale, and extend cognitive functioning (Reedy & Birren, 1980). By helping the elderly to bring past events back to mind and to relive, reexperience, and savor them, therapists can aid them in identifying and mitigating real guilt, in exorcising problematic childhood identifications, in resolving intense earlier conflicts, in reconciling family relationships, and in transmitting knowledge and values to others (Pincus, 1970). In addition, such therapy can help older persons integrate the aging experience into the entire life process and see death as a natural part of life.

"Everyday conversation is the primary mode through which people understand and account for their lives" (Bielby & Boden, 1981, p. 6). Life review is a way of redoing the past in the present through everyday conversation. Thus, life review therapy requires the ability to listen. By carefully listening as the older person relates and reconstructs the past by telling a life story, the therapist can begin to see and understand critical issues and unresolved conflicts, feelings of guilt over past mistakes or wrongdoings, concerns over inability as a parent, and other fears, anxieties, and doubts. The degree of emotion with which certain past events or people are recalled provides a clue as to the nature and intensity of feelings about them. Nuances and slips of the tongue can provide clues about self-image, the amount of stress one is experiencing, and the types of relationships the person hopes to foster. Listening intently also provides the opportunity to form interpersonal bonds with the older person and to reawaken the person's interests (Butler, 1961). Moreover, a sensitive listener can help the elderly put past events in proper perspective and turn the life review into "a positive attempt to reconcile life, to confront real guilt, and to find meaning in their lives, especially in the presence of acceptance and support from others" (Lewis & Butler, 1974, p. 169). Finally, the review of one's life with a concerned listener can allow one to see past mistakes in a new light and to deal with some of the guilt and fears related to them.

Lewis and Butler (1974) outline the following three steps in life review therapy:

1. *Recording of a detailed history.* This involves talking indepth to the older person about past life facts and events. It is an information-gathering, get-acquainted phase. The history taking may elicit memories of conflict and concern, thereby providing important diagnostic perceptions. To this end, a detailed oral history is preferable to a shorthand, computerized, or brief mental status assessment.

2. *Careful observation.* The therapist should carefully observe any emotional impact of memories, areas that are emphasized or deemphasized, and repetitious patterns of remembering. For example, if an individual with children provides an entire life history and never once mentions children, the therapist might infer that something is amiss in the family life area.

3. *Systematic eliciting of memories.* There are several techniques to elicit memories and help the older person successfully accomplish a life review. Lewis and Butler (1974) suggest the use of a written or taped autobiography; the individual is encouraged to write or tape record a detailed personal life story. To make contact with the life process through time and history, Dangott and Kalish (1979) suggest encouraging the person to remain playful in the life review, thus allowing for more creative movement. They also suggest that the "shaping events" of the person's life be recorded, basically answering the question: Which experiences have significantly shaped my life? They then recommend that the person go back and fill in the details of each event. The focus of the life review might be on the most important influences in the person's intellectual awakening and mental development, thinking back to teachers, parents, or friends or to an event, book, or poem. Dangott and Kalish (1979) also suggest dwelling on the particular events in the person's emotional development, asking, What have been the potent times of sorrow or loss in my life? What have been the disruptive experiences or events? They would encourage the person to remember important people who have had an influence, particularly those who have died. Finally, they suggest that the person record the deepest periods of joy, love, and sorrow and then remember and record the circumstances and surrounding details.

Reedy and Birren (1980) use a form of guided autobiography in life review therapy. They point out that:

historically, autobiography has been used in psychotherapy as a method of self help or self cure. For centuries autobiography has been used for 2 important therapeutic goals: As a confessional document to achieve catharsis and as a means to increase self insight and self discovery . . . autobiography is useful to increase self insight, elevate self esteem, generate feelings of pride, mastery, and self actualization, and reduce feelings of loneliness and social isolation. (p. 1)

In using a written or taped autobiography, it is important to pay careful attention to style, detail, and emphasis that may provide clues to various aspects of the person's life. What areas of life (family, work, leisure) are omitted? What pitch and tone of voice were used to discuss various people and events? The following specific aspects of the life review might be given special attention:

- *Pilgrimages.* Lewis and Butler (1974) encourage actual trips back to such important places as the place of birth, areas where childhood years were spent, homes of relatives, and other family places. The taking of photos and the collecting of newspaper articles or letters are to be encouraged on the pilgrimage.
- *Reunions.* Church, class, and family reunions help in the life review and might be encouraged.
- *Genealogy.* Tracing one's "roots" not only aids the life review but also helps one see one's proper place in time and history and allows one to gain a sense of other family members who have died. Lewis and Butler (1974) suggest the use of libraries, the family Bible, relatives, friends, cemeteries, and newspaper ads as valuable sources of information.
- *Memorabilia.* Scrapbooks, photo albums, old letters, and other such memorabilia are rich sources of memories.
- *Summation of life work.* A written or verbal work history, focusing particularly on one's contributions over the work life cycle, can play an important part in life review therapy, especially for those who valued work very highly.

Using these techniques, Reedy and Birren (1980) and Dangott and Kalish (1979) have used life review therapy successfully as a form of group therapy with the elderly. In working with the institutionalized elderly, Dangott and Kalish (1979) emphasize such questions as, What do you remember about where you grew up? What do you remember about parents, brothers, and sisters? How did you celebrate holidays and birthdays? Based on such questions, the group members can reminisce together around a particular theme. In this way, they can find atonement and self-forgiveness and discover new friends who share similar pasts.

Birren calls his method of life review group therapy "guided autobiography." He asks each member of the group to write an autobiography on a selected theme, such as family or work, and then to read and discuss the autobiography with the other members. Reedy and Birren (1980) conducted a pilot study using guided autobiographies from 45 elderly persons and found positive benefits from such therapy. The subjects were pretested and posttested using a variety of measures, such as the Leary Interpersonal

Checklist, the Speilberger State Trait Anxiety Scale, and the Treadway Mood Scale. After engaging in the therapy, the subjects showed greater self-acceptance, increases in energetic feelings and vigor, elevated moods, lower anxiety and tension, more positive views of others, and a sense of "social connectedness." Reedy and Birren (1980) concluded that sharing autobiographies in a group encourages "'developmental exchange,' the progressively deep, mutual exchange between individuals of personally important historical and emotional events. It is believed that such exchange activates the curative factors of self-understanding, catharsis, group cohesiveness, and a sense of the universality of lives" (p. 1).

It is thus particularly important that the therapist who chooses life review therapy as an intervention technique to help the troubled older person be an effective listener and be able to use the skills of exploration, focusing, and probing to help the individual order the past as a coherent whole (Pincus, 1970). The objective should be to help the troubled older person to achieve a sense of meaning and to maintain integrity over despair, thereby decreasing the risk of suicide.

REFERENCES

Bielby, D. D., & Boden, D. M. (1981, November). *The social production of life history: Doing the past.* Paper presented at the 34th annual meeting of the Gerontological Society of America, Toronto, Ontario, Canada.

Birren, J. E. (1964). *The psychology of aging.* Englewood, Cliffs, N.J.: Prentice-Hall.

Boylin, W., Gordon, S. K., & Nehrke, M. R. (1976). Reminiscing and ego integrity in institutionalized elderly males. *Gerontologist, 16*(2), 118–124.

Buhler, C. (1959). Theoretical observations about life's basic tendencies. *American Journal of Psychotherapy, 13*(3), 501–581.

Butler, R. N. (1961). Re-awakening interest. *Nursing Homes, 10,* 8–19.

Butler, R. N. (1963a). Recall in retrospection. *Journal of American Geriatrics Society, 11,* 523–529.

Butler, R. N. (1963b). The life review: An interpretation of reminiscence in the aged. *Psychiatry, 26*(1), 65–76.

Butler, R. N. (1964). The life review: An interpretation of reminiscence in the aged. In R. Kastenbaum (Ed.), *New thoughts on old age* (pp. 265–280). New York: Springer.

Butler, R. N. (1968). The life review: An interpretation of reminiscence in the aged. In B. Neugarten (Ed.), *Middle age and aging* (pp. 486–496). Chicago: University of Chicago Press.

Butler, R. N. (1971, 5). Age: The life review. *Psychology Today,* pp. 49–51, 89, 108.

Butler, R. N. (1980–1981). The life review: An unrecognized bonanza. *International Journal of Aging and Human Development, 12*(1), 35–38.

Coleman, P. G. (1974). Measuring reminiscence characteristics from conversation as adaptive features of old age. *International Journal of Aging and Human Development, 5*(3), 281–294.

Dangott, L. R., & Kalish, R. A. (1979). *A time to enjoy the pleasures of aging.* Englewood Cliffs, N. J.: Prentice-Hall.

Erikson, E. (1950). *Childhood and society.* New York: W. W. Norton.

Havighurst, R. J., & Glasser, R. (1972). An exploratory study of reminiscence. *Journal of Gerontology, 27* (2), 245–253.

Jung, C. G. (1934). *Modern man in search of a soul.* New York: Harcourt, Brace & Co.

Keen, S., & Fox, A. V. (1973). *Telling your story.* New York: Doubleday.

Kramer, C. H., Kramer, J., & Dunlop, H. E. (1966). Resolving grief. *Geriatric Nursing, 11,* 14–17.

Lewis, C. (1971). Reminiscing and self-concept in old age. *Journal of Gerontology, 26*(2), 240–243.

Lewis, M. L., & Butler, R. N. (1974). Life-review therapy: Putting memories to work in individual and group psychotherapy. *Geriatrics, 29*(11), 165–173.

Lieberman, M. A., & Falk, J. M. (1971). The remembered past as a source of research data for research on the life cycle. *International Journal of Aging and Human Development, 14,* 132–141.

McMahon, A. W., & Rhudick, P. J. (1967). Reminiscence in the aged: An adaptational response. In S. Levin & R. Kahana (Eds.), *Psychodynamic studies on aging: Creativity, reminiscing, and dying* (pp. 64–78). New York: International Universities Press.

Parkes, C. M. (1970). The first year of bereavement. *Psychiatry, 33,* 444–467.

Pincus, A. (1970). Reminiscence in aging and its implications for social work practice. *Social Work, 15*(3), 47–53.

Reedy, M. N., & Birren, J. E. (1980, September). *Life review through guided autobiography.* Paper presented at the annual meeting of the American Psychological Association, Montreal, Canada.

Romaniuk, M., & Romaniuk, J. (1981). Looking back: An analysis of reminiscence functions and triggers. *Experimental Aging Research, 7*(4), 477–489.

Chapter 9

Creative Therapy

Art is an organ of human life transmitting man's reasonable
perception into feeling.

Tolstoy

BACKGROUND

Although only fairly recently recognized as a treatment modality, creative
therapy—also referred to as arts therapy, creative arts therapy, expressive
therapy, or expression therapy—has its roots in prehistoric eras. "Our
predecessors expressed their relationship to animals and the world in cave
drawings, and sought the meaning of existence in imagery" (Wadeson, 1980,
p. 13). Dance, song, drama, and music have been a vital part of human
existence since man first attempted to placate the gods of nature with a
primitive dance of hops and skips around a fire (Shivers & Fait, 1980).
Primitive drama typically involved the entire community and combined
singing, dancing, shouting, clapping, playing of musical instruments, acrobat-
ics, mock use of weapons, and the wearing of costumes and masks. It was a
group expression of gaiety, revelry, and joy. Through the ages, art, music,
dance, and drama—which are primarily nonverbal—have been used as means
of communication and expression. Indeed, the arts may be considered
"humanity's oldest body of resources for expression and self realization"
(Anderson, 1977, p. ix). In creative therapies, the focus is on creativity, and
modalities are often combined.

The use of dance, song, drama, and visual arts in religious and magical
ways to cure physical or emotional ills is probably as old as art itself. Many
primitive tribes used elaborate artistic cures for physical diseases and
emotional disorders or to exorcise demons. Aristotle recognized the value of

dramatic play for relaxation "as a medicine" and noted the value of tragedy as catharsis because it allows for the "purgation of emotions" (Courtney, 1968, p. 10). Greek tragedies encouraged the expression of such emotions as pity and fear as the actors identified with characters.

St. Thomas Aquinas noted the value of drama for relaxation, and several early theorists focused on the therapeutic value of play, particularly dramatic play (Carr, 1902; Groos, 1976; Mitchell & Mason, 1948). Play is creative and fun, a safety valve for release of pent-up tensions and emotions, and it allows for spontaneity. In play, we temporarily forget our troubles and cares and relax. Play is refreshing and almost miraculously restores vitality. As Jonie Rhyne (1973), a leader in the field of art therapy, points out, "Art activity is a kind of play, underestimated even by Piaget" (p. 83). In play, the emphasis is on process, not product; the risk of failure is minimal; frustration is temporarily removed; and there is freedom and openness—all therapeutic characteristics (Fleshman & Fryrear, 1981).

The development of creative therapeutic intervention techniques with disturbed individuals has been closely allied with and greatly influenced by psychoanalysis and humanistic psychology. Freud (1955) and Jung (1964) placed great emphasis on symbolization, imagery, and the unconscious. Both recognized the therapeutic value of the drawing or painting of dreams, which are experienced as visual images and difficult to express in words. Jung in particular wrote extensively on the value of aesthetics and creativity, thus laying the basis for creative therapy. In this context, humanistic psychology—which emphasizes the importance of creativity, personal growth, and self-actualization and the attainment of one's full potential as a human being—provided additional impetus to the development and use of creative therapeutic intervention techniques.

The arts allow for creative expression, development of personal insight, and self-awareness. Similarly, spontaneity, flexibility, and originality resulting from the creative process are encouraged through the use of creative therapies. Art—whether in music, visual media, drama, or dance—is naturally therapeutic. It is a means of expanding the consciousness, of naturally becoming more aware of one's self, particularly of the connection between mind and body. It forces us to become more in tune with our senses (sight, hearing, touch) and our bodies. As creative expression, art provides a healthy, natural outlet for feelings and emotions. As Durland (1978) points out, "One purpose of creative drama is to open the mind so one may enter into the creative world of imagination and discover that which is unique and lies within us" (p. 138). Drama as a therapeutic technique naturally results in insight, self-awareness, and self-discovery—processes that psychoanalysis also aims to stimulate.

The arts also provide a means to achieve an identity. The search for identity—one's sense of who one is and where one stands in relation to God, the universe, and other humans—has always led to music, art, and drama. "The need for self-relation, direction, and life enhancement drives people to search for individuality . . . rather than to remain a part of the mass society" (Arnold, 1976, p. 1). Nowhere can one find a better opportunity to develop and express one's unique individuality and identity than through participation in drawing, painting, sculpting, music, drama, or dance.

Thus, creative therapy offers the elderly a valuable means of self-expression, insight, and self-awareness through free association and imagery. It engages the elderly individual in the creative process, encouraging spontaneity, flexibility, and emotional expression. It is also a valuable means of releasing fear and doubt, guilt and grief—emotions that plague many potentially suicidal elderly; and it provides a positive experience of participation in a social group, with accompanying feelings of acceptance and belonging, self-esteem and self-concept, and personal competence, mastery, and accomplishment. Finally, since most forms of creative therapy utilize some form of reminiscence and life review, it offers the additional benefits available from those techniques.

In this vein, Lucas (1964) sees "the need for definite and positive programs in the field of gerontology, based not solely upon the concept of security for the aged, but, more importantly, on programs that build for the older citizen an atmosphere of creativity and belonging" (p. 5). Similarly, Simone de Beauvoir (1972) noted that "old age exposes the failure of our entire civilization. There is only one solution if old age is not to be an absurd parody of our former life, and that is to go on pursuing ends that give our existence meaning—devotion to individuals, to groups, or to causes, social, political, intellectual, or to creative work" (p. 18).

In this chapter, we describe the benefits of four creative therapies—art, music, dance, and drama—and the particular creative therapeutic techniques that have been used effectively with the elderly. Special attention is given to creative dramatics, a therapeutic intervention that we have used successfully with the elderly. We suggest that all of the therapeutic interventions described be implemented with the assistance of a specialist in art, music, dance, or drama therapy.

ART THERAPY

Art therapy—involving drawing, painting, clay modeling, sculpting, metal art, and other forms of visual, graphic, or plastic art—has its roots in psychoanalytic psychology. What is impossible to adequately express or describe in words, one can paint or draw. Thus, in the context of dreaming, Freud noted that:

> we experience it [a dream] predominately in visual images; feelings may be present too, and thoughts interwoven as well; the other senses may also experience something, but nonetheless it is predominately a question of images. Part of the difficulty of giving an account of dreams is due to our having to translate the images into words. "I could draw it," a dreamer often says to us, "but I don't know how to say it." (Wadeson, 1980, p. 210)

The nonverbal form of communication in painting or drawing allows one to express thoughts, feelings, and emotions vividly and personally in images and symbols. The free choice of colors and types of paper or materials further enhances expression, uniqueness, and individuality. One can draw anger or rage, pain or sadness, choosing appropriate lines and strokes or colors that signify these moods and feelings. Working with clay or fingerpaints is particularly effective. One can actually squeeze, push, and physically manipulate the substance. In short, art therapy gives disturbed individuals the opportunity to "listen with their eyes" (Landgarten, 1981, p. 4). The senses are aroused and stimulated as one sees and touches.

In general, the benefits claimed for art therapy are of three types: psychoanalytic, creative, and existential/humanistic. Margaret Naumberg (1950), a pioneer in the field, emphasized the psychoanalytic role of art therapy, claiming that art represents "symbolic speech" (p. 18). She regarded the translation of visual symbols (considered to result from repression) as the basis of psychoanalysis. In other words, art permits the direct expression of dreams, fantasies, and other inner experiences; and the pictured projections of unconscious material speeds up the therapeutic process. Similarly, Kramer (1958) noted the value of art as a means of sublimation, allowing the client to act out forbidden impulses symbolically through visual images. She advocated art as a creative therapeutic medium, stressing the healing quality of the process of creation:

> Art is a means of widening the range of human experiences by creating equivalents for such experiences. It is an area wherein experiences can be chosen, varied, repeated at will. In the creative act, conflict is re-experienced, resolved and integrated . . . . The arts throughout history have helped man to reconcile the eternal conflict between the individual's instinctual urges and the demands of society . . . . The process of sublimation constitutes the best way to deal with a basic human dilemma, but the conflicting demands of

superego and id cannot be permanently reconciled.... In the artistic product conflict is formed and contained but only partly neutralized. The artist's position epitomizes the precarious human situation: while his craft demands the greatest self-discipline and perseverance, he must maintain access to the primitive impulses and fantasies that constitute the raw material for his creative work.

The art therapist makes creative experiences available to disturbed persons in the service of the total personality; he must use methods compatible with the inner laws of artistic creation.... His primary function is to assist the process of sublimation, an act of integration and synthesis which is performed by the ego, wherein the peculiar fusion between reality and fantasy, between the unconscious and the conscious, which we call art is reached. (pp. 6–23)

Those who focus on the existential and humanistic values of art therapy emphasize the development of spontaneity, flexibility, self-expression, and originality and of relationships with others through group or family art sessions. Art is viewed as a way of expressing feelings about self, the world, and human relationships. For example, Dwedney (1977) describes the following techniques that have been used with the elderly in the Ontario Psychiatric Hospital in London:

- *Drawing and coloring an object from observation.* In this exercise, the elderly individual chooses some object such as a cup and draws it. This gives the individual a better sense of reality.
- *Picture completion.* Here, a picture of a person or an object cut from a magazine is put on a page and the elderly individual completes the background. This encourages the use of imagination, skill, and originality.

Landgarten (1981) has effectively used the following techniques with the elderly:

- *Symbolization of events and emotions.* The elderly individual is asked to draw, sculpt, or otherwise express certain events and their attending emotions that have been experienced during the week. The art work is then discussed with the therapist or others in the art therapy group.
- *Positive lifetime review.* The elderly individual is asked to create scenes from the past (place, job, family) or to make a pictorial album showing aspects of past life.

- *Positive aspects of leisure.* The individual draws a symbol designating the positive aspects of not being busy or draws or pastes pictures of various leisure-time activities.

- *Unfinished messages.* Individuals make a collage to depict family, friends, or acquaintances and things left unsaid. This technique is particularly valuable for elderly persons who are facing death and may need to express unsaid feelings and messages to reduce guilt.

- *Depiction of one's partner.* The elderly pair off and draw their partners, then discuss the drawings.

- *The who-you-are box.* Individuals decorate the outside of a box showing who they are. Inside they put pictures, drawings, or physical items representing things about themselves. This exercise reveals how one feels about one's self and shows the important attributes, past or present talents or accomplishments, and important people, places, and things in one's life.

- *Depiction of problems.* The elderly individual is asked to draw some of the problems the elderly throughout the world face. This technique allows for recognition and acceptance of failing health, loss of mobility, death, and other concerns of the elderly.

Art therapy has proven to be particularly effective for chronic pain patients. The expression of pain and the accompanying feelings of anger, rage, guilt, or sorrow through artwork permits catharsis and leads to the successful management of the feeling (Landgarten, 1981). Wadeson (1980), who has used art therapy with suicidal patients with positive results, notes that suicidal individuals have strong pent-up emotions, particularly anger, that are often stored up over a lifetime. Art therapy provides a method of communication in which to express such suicidal ideations. The release of such feelings in symbols through artwork can provide a suitable nonviolent way of enacting them. Many elderly also experience feelings of depression, and artwork is one method of working through such feelings. Such feelings, expressed through art, can then be shared and discussed with positive results. Finally, suicidal individuals can obtain therapeutic benefits by examining their own feelings and emotions as expressed in concrete form in art works.

MUSIC THERAPY

Aristotle believed that music had the power to change the soul. Indeed music has been referred to as the universal language. As Arnold (1976) defines it, "music is the organization of sounds, sounds that express meaning, hold significance to the listener, draw reactions, or provoke thought and contemplation" (p. 97). In primitive society, inner emotions were expressed through song and dance, which also served as communication bonds between people (Arnold, 1976).

Music is the oldest form of art to be associated with the cure of the sick. In primitive tribes, songs, chants, and dances were performed to cure the sick. The ancient Greeks and Egyptians similarly believed in the curative powers of music. Numerous accounts of music being used to cure the sick can also be found in the literature of the eighteenth, nineteenth, and twentieth centuries. However, clinical interest in music as therapy appeared only shortly after World War I, when music was used therapeutically with hospitalized veterans. Thereafter, the power of music to alter moods and change behavior gained wide formal recognition.

Music therapy involves "having music in the environment, such as background music, actively listening to music, or making music" (Fleshman & Fryrear, 1981, p. 59). It uses music to "provide inspiration, alter mood, stimulate memories and discussion, or to accompany physical movement or dance" (Fleshman & Fryrear, 1981, p. 59).

The major techniques of music therapy involve observation, participation, and creation. Observation involves listening to music or watching a musical performance. The listening or watching is active, involving the mind and senses, requiring attention, concentration, and involvement of the participant. For example, the music of Mahler has been effectively used to evoke certain emotions and moods, such as sadness and somberness (F. Wells, 1977). The participation may be through humming, singing, foot tapping, clapping, swaying or rocking to the music, dancing, or engaging in other body movements. The playing of musical instruments or involvement in a rhythm band, using cymbals, bells, tambourines, drums, or other percussion instruments, is also participatory. Most participation occurs in a group situation. Group singing and dancing with others are common favorites. Music creation involves writing, composing, or otherwise making music. In any event, music is rhythmic and structured, a natural form of organization. Thus, F. Wells (1977) stresses the importance of using our own bodies to create sounds and thereby become part of the music, that is, the music is us.

Musical participation evokes powerful associations and moods and encourages nonverbal expression of thought, feelings, and emotions. Through participation in or creation of one's own song, dance, or melody, self-expression, self-awareness, and creativity are enhanced. Specifically, Gaston (1968) cites the following benefits of musical therapy. It provides or evokes:

- experience within structure, that is, time-ordered behavior
- ability-ordered behavior, according to physical and psychological response levels

- affectively ordered behavior
- sensory-elaborated behavior
- self-expression
- compensatory endeavors for the handicapped individual
- opportunities for socially acceptable rewards and nonrewards
- enhancement of pride in self by providing for successful experiences and the feeling of being needed by others
- experience for relating to others
- verbal and nonverbal social interaction and communication
- cooperation and competition in socially acceptable forms
- entertainment and recreation necessary to the general therapeutic environment
- learning of realistic social skills and personal behavior patterns acceptable in institutional and community peer groups

Others have identified particular benefits and advantages to be derived from music therapy:

- It can be a source of gratification and personal accomplishment and growth (Schneider, Unkefer, & Gaston, 1968).
- It is a means of expressing tender emotions, such as love and loyalty (Schneider et al., 1968).
- It is a major form of nonverbal communication (Schneider et al., 1968).
- It enables one to utilize rhythm to energize and motivate (Gaston, 1968).
- It stimulates the mind, relaxes the body, and comforts the spirit (Bright, 1972).
- It has soothing qualities that promote relaxation, unblock the mind, and encourage free association (Bright, 1972).
- It has memory-invoking properties (Bright, 1972).
- It offers a powerful mechanism of "psychocatharsis" to evoke emotions and associations and allow one to "get things out of the system" through tears and expressions of fear and guilt (Bright, 1972, p. 15; Fleshman & Fryrear, 1981; Rathbone & Lucas, 1970, p. 182; F. Wells, 1977).
- It provides an avenue of shared experience, interest, and activities, thus promoting friendship, group participation, and social bonds (Bright, 1972).

Many practitioners have used music therapy effectively with the elderly (Boxberger & Cotter, 1968; Browne & Winkelmayer, 1968; Cotter, 1960;

Gaston, 1968; Kurz, 1960; Roth, 1961; A. Wells, 1954). The elderly particularly enjoy group singing, piano and guitar music, rhythm bands, and the music of an earlier era that invokes pleasant reminiscences of childhood days, early courtship experiences, and other significant life events. Thus, music therapy has been used with the elderly as an outlet for creative expression, as a vehicle to invoke powerful emotions, and as an aid in grief work and in dealing with the experience of death and dying. It naturally encourages group participation and, as such, has reportedly alleviated feelings of loneliness, hopelessness, depression, and despair in elderly participants. Finally, in music therapy, improvements in breathing, posture, muscle tone, and physical health in general have been noted, especially when the therapy involves dance and other forms of bodily movement.

DANCE THERAPY

Dance and music are intricately related; dance is music set to motion. Predating the spoken word, dance is thought to be the very first means of human communication. Primitive people attributed mystical and magical powers to dance, engaging in war dances, rain dances, ghost dances, and religious or ritualistic dances. Joy, fear, hope, and awe were all expressed through dance.

"Dance and movement arts bind the individual together physically, mentally, and psychologically. In this art form, the individual uses the most primary means of self expression and communication—his/her body" (Fleshman & Fryrear, 1981, p. 91). In dance, all of the senses are used and basic rhythms of life are employed—breathing, the heartbeat, muscular tension, and relaxation (Fleshman & Fryrear, 1981).

Arnold (1976) has defined dance as:

> a spontaneous or artistic (constructed) movement or series of movements that is an expressed reaction to an intrinsic or extrinsic stimulus. According to this definition, dance may be movement for the joy of moving, reacting, and responding or it may be movement deliberately constructed to express thought or to display some perception of a choreographer. (p. 71)

More precisely, Arnold (1976) cites the dictionary definition of dance as:

> rhythmic movement having as its aim the creation of visual designs by a series of poses and tracing of patterns through space in the course of measured units of time, the two components, static and kinetic, receiving varying emphasis (as in ballet, natya, and modern

dance) and being executed by different parts of the body in accordance with temperament, artistic percepts, and purpose. (p. 71)

Thus, through dance, physical impulses and internal psychological states and feelings are released in bodily movement.

Dance as a form of therapeutic intervention has its basis in the development of the modern dance. Isadora Duncan was the first dancer to revive expressive, natural dance as a way to live more fully and freely. She derived her philosophy of modern dance from her understanding of dance in classical Greece.

Chace (1953), one of the earliest practitioners of dance therapy, viewed it as:

the specific use of dance movements as a means of nonverbal communication, emotional release of both hostile and tender feelings, physical relaxation, and increased self-awareness. Therapeutically, the beauty of perfection of the dance movements is not to be given primary consideration. Instead, the dance therapist interprets the patient's movements as a communication of his individual emotions, mood of the moment, and degree of security. The development of the ability to dance well, gracefully, and with good coordination and skill is subordinate to the needs of the patients.

Because disruption in communication is the important problem for the psychiatric patient, dance therapy provides the individual with a means of reestablishing communication with his personal and social environment when he is otherwise cut off by the patterns of his illness. (p. 34)

Thus, dance therapy is a psychotherapeutic technique that uses bodily movement as a means to express repressed feelings, thoughts, and emotions, to bring the unconscious to conscious awareness, and to further the emotional, mental, and physical integration of the person. The aims of dance therapy are threefold: physical, psychological, and social:

The physical goals may include the stimulation and energizing of the patients' bodies in free, natural movement; the releasing of physical tension through activity and relaxation exercises; the building up and increasing of individual ability to perform the motor acts of daily living with easy coordination; and the broadening of the patient's movement repertoire. The psychological goals may include stimulating and encouraging patients to express themselves freely in movement; channeling self-expression into meaningful dance forms; helping patients adjust to a world of reality; and aiding the development of new skills and interest so that the patient's attention is removed from his own symptoms. Social goals of the dance therapist may include getting the patients to join a group activity that would develop its own goals; developing personal and social relationships in a recreational situation; and encouraging interpersonal relationships. (Fleshman & Fryrear, 1981, pp. 82–83)

Dance therapy is body talk, as contrasted with other talk therapies. Its techniques emphasize spontaneous, expressive body movements, ranging from simple swaying to and fro to elaborately patterned ballroom dancing. Chace (1953) used a circle formation to encourage group participation. Flexibility, spontaneity, and creativity were encouraged in order to release tension, allow for emotional expression, and provide relaxation. Chace stressed that the dance motions should have a reaching-out quality to ensure acceptance. Touching was encouraged, but only when the individual freely initiated it. Rosen (1957), another leading dance therapist, has emphasized the need for at least one assistant in the sessions and cited the value of live piano accompaniment, which allows for varied rhythms, melody and flexibility. Swinging, swaying, sliding, and gliding are all acceptable techniques.

According to Wapner (1981), a successful program of dance therapy should include the following movements of a dance repertoire: walking, sliding, gliding, hopping, jumping, jogging, turning, crawling, and rolling. Bending and stretching, the use of stylized and creative movements, expressions of all sorts, exercises, and rhythmic movement are all encouraged. Folk-dancing, tap-dancing, square-dancing, and ballroom dancing may also be used. The elderly particularly enjoy dances from their young adult days; many have participated in folk- or square-dance clubs during their lives.

Chace (1953) has reported the results of a study of the effects of a dance therapeutic intervention with schizophrenics. Projective tests were administered to the group before and after participation in 21 dance therapy sessions. Pretests and posttests were also given to a matched control group. After participation in the dance therapy, the patients showed marked improvement in body image, while decreases or no improvement were noted for controls. The movements and energy levels of the patients in dance therapy also increased markedly.

Dance therapy has also been used successfully with emotionally disturbed children (Anderson, 1977; Bartenieff, 1958; Bender & Boas, 1941; Bunzel, 1948; Chace, 1953), with the mentally retarded (Arje & Berryman, 1966; F. Robins & J. Robins, 1965), and with emotionally disturbed, mentally ill adults (Goldstein, Lingas, & Sheafor, 1965) to release physical tension and express emotions and thus to achieve catharsis and to induce relaxation, social interaction, and group participation.

These studies indicate that dance can heighten mind/body awareness and provide for improved body image and self-concept. It can provide an effective means of personal expression and individuality. Through creative dance, disturbed individuals are able to express fantasies, hidden thoughts, and disturbing emotions, and deal with conflicts. Anderson (1977) has noted that dance increases one's movement repertoire and, as a result, one's space to be or physical self. Dance is fun and allows for an immediate physical expression of joy. Laughter is a frequent occurrence in dance therapy sessions; and many come away from such sessions feeling loose, full of energy, relaxed, and refreshed. There is also a sense of power and mastery that comes from exercising the body and mind through movement and dance.

Older people may experience all of these benefits from movement and dance therapy. Such therapy is particularly beneficial for the old who are experiencing physical decline and decreased mobility. Garnet (1974) has effectively used movement sequences that employ rhythmic use of swings, twists, stretches, pulls, and pushes to meet physical needs and stimulate somatic and psychological feelings of comfort, ease, and humor in elderly subjects. Merritt (1971) has used dance therapy to help elderly patients adjust physically, mentally, emotionally, and socially to their nursing home. The patients gained self-confidence and prided themselves on their ability to respond to the music. Dance therapy with the elderly can also be used effectively to elicit memories of the past and to encourage social participation, thus alleviating feelings of isolation and depression.

CREATIVE DRAMATICS

Background

"If he is indeed wise he does not bid you enter the house of his wisdom, but rather leads you to the threshold of your own mind." This quotation from *The Prophet* (Gibran, 1977, p. 56) beautifully expresses the theory behind creative dramatics. A relatively new form of dramatic art, creative dramatics is a form of spontaneous creation and expression of feelings drawing upon both past life experiences and feelings and emotions of the moment. No particular skills or talents are required to participate in creative dramatics.

All that is required is imagination and a wealth of life experiences and feelings.

Creative dramatics involves motion and rhythm, color and visual experiences, storytelling and acting, pantomime, and improvisation. It was first introduced with children as a way to tap imagination and creativity and allow for self-exploration, emotional release, and fun. The technique permits a continual discovery of ideas, thoughts, memories, talents, sayings, songs, colors, words, people, feelings, and sounds. Because it is for the moment, it is constantly changing, developing, and combining, meeting the needs of the group on a specific day, at a given time. As participatory drama, it is created with and by the members of the group; therefore no final product is expected or required, other than that discovered or explored at the moment. As a form of participatory theatre, it emphasizes the process of *doing* drama, of actually creating images, scenes, and dialogue rather than merely producing a polished, memorized piece. Such an art form provides a "fail-safe" experience that can be successfully participated in by the educated and uneducated, young and old, alike.

As a therapeutic technique, creative dramatics has its roots in dramatic play and is closely related to psychodrama. Play has long been recognized as essential to the normal, healthy development of children. According to Courtney (1968), "dramatic play is a reflection of the child's unconscious . . . . The content of dramatic play is unconscious symbolic thought based on experience. The purpose of play is to reproduce in symbolic form the unsolved experiences of life and attempt solutions" (p. 273).

Psychodrama grew out of Jacob Moreno's experience with Viennese children at play. Derived from the Greek terms *psyche*, meaning mind or soul, and *dramein*, meaning to do or to act, psychodrama refers to the doing or acting of thoughts and emotions through speech, gestures, and movement (Duke, 1974). It is "a group psychotherapy process during which individuals spontaneously enact elements and events from their own lives" (Fleshman & Fryrear, 1981, p. 48). In psychodrama, individuals play roles and create parts; the emphasis is on spontaneity, creativity, action, process, self-disclosure, risk taking and the here-and-now (Moreno, 1934). The individual acts out unconscious thoughts, feelings, and impulses in order to recapitulate unsolved problems and experience catharsis. The group drama encourages empathy as the players identify with one another. Like psychodrama, creative dramatics involves role creation and role playing, improvisation, mime and pantomime, storytelling and enactment, and a variety of other therapeutic techniques.

In the last decade, creative dramatics has been used increasingly with the elderly. The American Theatre Association first became involved with adult theatre in 1973 when Vera Mowry Roberts, then the association's president, asked Paul Kozelka to chair the association's first committee on theatre for retirees. Since that time, senior theatre groups have sprung up all over the country. The Living Stage in Washington, D.C., involves seniors in improvisation theatre. Ruth Tate directs a group of seniors in White Plains, New York, that has won numerous awards in local theatre competitions. The Amber Area Arts Alliance of Amber, Pennsylvania, sponsors a project called Third Age Theatre, a comprehensive dramatics program for individuals over age 55. A group called the College Avenue Players, comprising adults ranging in age from 68 to 85, has performed new plays for thousands of people throughout the East Bay area. A large number of such theatre groups, comprised totally of elderly players, were represented at meetings on the arts held by the NCOA in January, 1978.

In 1973, the National Council on the Aging (NCOA) created a special division called the Center on Arts and Aging. The division's purpose is to activate local and national groups to consider the important role the arts can play in life enrichment for the elderly.

Techniques and Benefits

Creative dramatic techniques that have been used effectively with the elderly include:

- *Pantomime.* The portrayal of feelings through expressions and body movement; charades is an example.
- *Improvisation.* The creation of scripts and dialogues using spontaneous expression and movement, the main purpose of which is to "warm up" actors, break down self-consciousness, and start imaginations working. The actors pretend to be inanimate objects, other persons, food, and so on.
- *Intergenerational theatre.* The involvement of children and the elderly together in the dramatization of themes, stories, and books.
- *Creative writing.* Imaginative sentence completions; creation of stories, dialogue, and scripts.
- *Group poetry.* Original poetry created and written together in a group.
- *Talking book series.* Oral/visual projects in which children's books are transposed into radio scripts accompanied by acetate drawings and shown with the use of an overhead projector.
- *Movement.* Interpretive dance, exercise, and other physical involvement using the senses and various parts of the body.
- *Visual art.* Creation of book covers, acetate drawings, props, and scenery for use in intergenerational theatre scenes.

- *Oral history theatre.* Personal stories transposed into scripts for the stage for purposes of sharing and discussion. Oral history theatre can embrace the collective works of the elder person, illustrating life experiences, important historical moments, and day-to-day living. There may be as many oral history pieces as there are individual stories. The storyteller contributes a talent, a life experience; the participants contribute their own dialogue; and the group becomes united through the "suspension of disbelief" as they reenact the story.

- *Vaudeville or variety show.* A show consisting of original sketches, parodies of current TV programs, or popular songs with new lyrics that refer to local personalities or events. Groups can have a great time with a minimum of rehearsal by dramatizing jokes or acting out cartoons from magazines and newspapers. Skits and sing-alongs may also be included.

- *Play reading.* Actors perform with script-in-hand readings of appropriate plays for their own pleasure or for an audience.

Creative drama provides many benefits for elderly participants. Czurles (1969) has noted that "age does not stop creative growth, its satisfactions, and developmental values. On the contrary, it frees the individual for the maximum personal involvement. The arts can help the elderly lead increasingly enriching lives". Based on his own experience, Nolter (1973) offers support for the use of creative dramatic techniques with the elderly: "Older persons should become involved in dramatics because it is an immediate creative experience which gives internal and external satisfaction" (p. 153).

From data she collected on the effects of drama on the elderly, Gray (1974) cited the following as the major benefits: opportunity to be of service to others, increased self-confidence resulting from successful memorization and good performance, communication and social interaction skills developed through the group experience, and the emotional outlet provided by the experience. Burger (1980), Clark (1978), Clark and Osgood (in press), and others have demonstrated that the elderly who participate in the creative drama experience can change their lives. Many of them begin to communicate and see themselves as useful again; life takes on new meaning. Other practitioners working with the elderly in creative dramatics programs across the country have cited such benefits as improved memory; increased verbal and cognitive skills; improved communication; increased socialization; improved group skills; improved sense of self and self-esteem; achievement of emotional outlets; greater creative expression; improvement in expressing originality; greater self-discovery and personal mastery; achievement of new sources of joy and pleasure; healthier, more meaningful recreation and leisure time; and the achievement of status, prestige, and self-fulfillment that were formerly acquired through work and family involvement (Duke, 1974;

Sunderland, 1976; Vorenberg, 1979; Way, 1967). In addition, oral history as a form of reminiscence provides all the benefits cited earlier. Finally, the dramatization of social issues, such as death and poverty, and medical problems by the elderly participants in the theatre group enables them to come to terms and deal with them.

A Case Study

In a recent study of the impact of participation by the elderly in creative drama, Clark and Osgood (in press) selected 103 elderly at seven nutrition sites in Richmond, Virginia, and Northern Virginia to participate for 10 months in weekly creative drama sessions led by a trained drama expert. A matched control group of 27 persons (matched on age, race, sex, marital status, income, and health) was chosen for comparison purposes.

The drama groups ranged in size from 3 to 25 persons. Each group met weekly and engaged in improvisation, radio drama, oral history theatre, intergenerational theatre, group poetry, movement, visual art work, and other creative dramatic techniques. The participants and nonparticipants were pretested and posttested using a global question on life satisfaction, together with questions assessing perceptions of health, loneliness, and subjective age identification. To assess life satisfaction, the subjects were asked to respond to the following item: Overall, how satisfied are you with your life? The response choices were satisfied and not satisfied. To measure loneliness, the subjects were asked, How often do you feel lonely? The response choices included most of the time, much of the time, some of the time, hardly ever, and never. Subjective age identification was assessed by asking the subjects, How do you see yourself as far as age goes? The response choices included old, middle-aged, and young.

Pretest and posttest data were computer analyzed using analysis-of-change scores (Campbell & Stanley, 1963) to determine whether or not members of the experimental group changed significantly more on the three measures than did members of the control group after participation in the program. To calculate change scores, the mean scores at Time 1 were subtracted from the mean scores at Time 2 for both experimental and control groups and the change in means was calculated for each group. A one-tailed t test of differences in changed means was then applied to test for statistical significance of change from Time 1 to Time 2. The study also included qualitative analyses of excerpts from diaries kept by the drama leader and the participants, interviews with the participants, and systematically recorded observations of group sessions, anecdotes, and individual case studies.

The quantitative analysis-of-change scores revealed significant changes on major dependent variables. Compared to those in the control group, the participants in the experimental group improved considerably on life satisfaction, loneliness, and subjective age identification from Time 1 to Time 2. After 10 months, the participants in the creative drama program were happier and more satisfied with life in general, and they perceived themselves as less lonely and younger than members of the control group. When all experimental subjects were compared with controls, the change in subjective age identification from Time 1 to Time 2 was not statistically significant. However, when only those participants from the five sites in Northern Virginia who had worked with the experienced drama expert were compared to the control subjects, the difference from Time 1 to Time 2 was statistically significant. Table 9–1 displays results of the quantitative analyses. All results are significant at or above the .05 level of probability.

Qualitative analyses of recorded observations, excerpts from the diaries of drama leaders and participants, and interviews with participants revealed that those who took part in the creative drama program opened up and expressed feelings, became close as a group, and made friendships that they carried out of the drama sessions. The participants became more and more comfortable with each other as the sessions continued. They opened up and expressed

---

Table 9–1 Quantitative Results of Participation by Elderly in Creative Drama Program

Mean Scores on Global Measure of Life Satisfaction

Group:	Time 1	Time 2
Experimental	.84	.97
Control	.87	.92
	t (106) – 1.85, p = < .03	

Mean Scores on Loneliness

Group:	Time 1	Time 2
Experimental	2.7	2.3
Control	2.4	2.4
	t(54) = 1.91, p = < .03	

Mean Scores on Subjective Age-Identification

Group:	Time 1	Time 2
Experimental	1.9	2.1
Control	1.9	1.9
	t(54) = 2.83, p = < .01	

Source: From *Seniors on Stage* by P. A. Clark and N. J. Osgood, in press, New York: Praeger Publishers. Copyright 1985 by Praeger Publishers. Reprinted with permission.

feelings, they learned to cooperate and work together as a group, they laughed a lot, and they gained enough self-confidence to perform in front of others. Some with psychiatric problems opened up and came out of their withdrawn states during the course of the project. Many of them noted, either through written or verbal comments, improvements in their outlook on life, in how they felt physically and mentally, in their personal lives, and in their relations with family and friends. They experienced joy and excitement and in general became happier, better functioning human beings.

The following excerpts from the leaders' diaries illustrate some of the changes that occurred as a result of the 10-month experience:

- One participant who was confined to a wheelchair and who had danced as a youth participated in the group as a handicapped dancer and was overjoyed by the experience.

- Another participant was under psychiatric care for extreme depression when she joined the drama group. She reported that her participation in the oral history theatre had enabled her to understand some of the past events in her life and to put them in perspective. In the course of the 10 months, this participant just blossomed as she became more expressive, less withdrawn, and happier.

- Another woman was severely depressed and confused when she joined the drama sessions. Before participating, she had been ignored by fellow members at the site. When she started participating, the members of the drama group talked to her and took an active interest in her, helping her with her script work and memorization. As a result of this attention, she became more sociable and responded openly, verbally and physically, to the others.

- Most participants at the various sites had not interacted with each other as individuals before the drama group was formed. After the group formed, the members became friends and interacted with each other on a regular basis at the centers outside the group. In general, they became much more active and sociable as a result of their participation.

- Before the study began, all of the sites were cut off from intergenerational contact. The introduction of children into the sites had a very positive effect on the elderly participants. They became much more physically and verbally expressive, more animated (smiling, laughing, touching), happier, and more enthusiastic.

The following quotations from the participants illustrate how they personally perceived the impact of participation in drama on their lives:

- "It gives me a little pleasure out of life." (septuagenarian at one site)
- "I think it's kept me on my toes and interested." (77-year-old participant who credited his recovery from a recent heart attack to his experience in creative dramatics)
- "It has carried me back into the world again." (aged participant)

In the kind of complex, fast-moving, ever-changing society we live in, we need more than ever before to develop creative expression. Flexibility, adaptability, and innovation are the keys to our survival. The creative arts can help to develop these attributes in older individuals, thus better preparing them to cope with the losses, problems, and stresses of aging and to adapt successfully to late life.

REFERENCES

Anderson, W. (Ed.). (1977). *Therapy and the arts: Tools of consciousness.* New York: Harper & Row.

Arje, F. B., & Berryman, D. (1966). New help for the severely retarded and emotionally disturbed child. *Journal of Rehabilitation, 32,* 14–15, 67.

Arnold, N. (1976). *The interrelated arts in leisure: Perceiving and creating.* St. Louis, Mo.: C. V. Mosby Co.

Bartenieff, I. (1958). How is the dancing teacher equipped to do dance therapy? In E. T. Gaston (Ed.), *Music therapy* (pp. 145–150). Lawrence, Kans.: Allen Press.

Bender, L., & Boas, F. (1941). Creative dance in therapy. *American Journal of Orthopsychiatry, 11,* 235–245.

Boxberger, R., & Cotter, V. W. (1968). Music therapy for geriatric patients. In E. T. Gaston (Ed.), *Music in therapy* (pp. 271–280). New York: Macmillan.

Bright, R. (1972). *Music in geriatric care.* New York: St. Martins Press.

Browne, H. E., & Winkelmayer, R. (1968). A structured music therapy program in geriatrics. In E. T. Gaston (Ed.), *Music in therapy* (pp. 281–293). New York: Macmillan.

Bunzel, G. (1948). Psychokinetics and dance therapy. *Journal of Health and Physical Education, 19,* 180–181.

Burger, I. (1980). *Creative drama for senior adults.* Wilton, Conn.: Morehouse-Barlow.

Campbell, D. T., & Stanley, J. C. (1963). Experimental and quasiexperimental designs for research. In N. L. Gage (Ed.), *Handbook of research and teaching* (pp. 171–246). Chicago: Rand McNally.

Carr, H. H. (1902). *The survival of play.* Report of investigation for the University of Colorado, Department of Psychology and Education.

Chace, M. (1953). Dance as an adjunctive therapy with hospitalized mental patients. *Bulletin of the Menninger Clinic, 17,* 219–225.

Clark, P. (1978). *Theater arts and the aging.* Unpublished master's thesis, Virginia Commonwealth University, Richmond, Va.

Clark, P., & Osgood, N. J. (in press). *Seniors on stage: The impact of applied theatre on the elderly.* New York: Praeger Press.

Cotter, V. W. (1960). *Effects of the use of music on the behavior of geriatric patients.* Unpublished master's thesis, University of Kansas, Lawrence, Kans.

Courtney, R. (1968). *Play, drama, and thought: The intellectual background of drama in education.* New York: Drama Book Publishers.

Czurles, S. A. (1969, June). *Enriching retirement living through the arts.* Paper presented at a seminar on Enlightening Retirement Living Through the Arts at Union College, Schenectady, N. Y.

de Beauvoir, S. (1972). *The coming of age.* New York: G. P. Putnam's Sons.

Duke, C. (1974). *Creative dramatics and English teaching.* Urbana, Ill.: National Council of Teachers of English.

Durland, F. C. (1978). *Creative dramatics for children.* Kent, Ohio: Kent State University Press.

Dwedney, I. (1977). An art therapy program for geriatric patients. In E. Ulman & P. Dachinger (Eds.), *Art therapy in theory and practice* (2nd ed., pp. 126–131). New York: Schocken Books.

Fleshman, B., & Fryrear, J. (1981). *The arts in therapy.* Chicago: Nelson Hall.

Freud, S. (1955). *Origin and development of psychoanalysis.* Chicago: Regnery-Gateway.

Garnet, E. D. (1974). A movement therapy for older people. *Dance Therapy: Focus on Dance, 7,* 59–61.

Gaston, E. T. (Ed.). (1968). *Music in therapy.* New York: Macmillan.

Gibran, K. (1977). *The prophet.* New York: Alfred A. Knopf, Inc.

Goldstein, C., Lingas, C., & Sheafor, D. (1965). Interpretative or creative movement as a sublimation tool in music therapy. *Journal of Music Therapy, 2,* 11–15.

Groos, K. (1976). *The play of man* (E. L. Baldwin, Trans.). New York: Arno Press.

Jung, C. G. (1964). *Man and his symbols.* Garden City, N.Y.: Doubleday.

Kramer, E. (1958). *Art therapy in a children's community.* Springfield, Ill.: Charles C Thomas.

Kurz, C. E. (1960). *The effects of a planned music program on the day hall sound level and personal appearance of geriatric patients.* Unpublished master's thesis, University of Kansas. Lawrence, Kans.

Landgarten, H. B. (1981). *Clinical art therapy: A comprehensive guide.* New York: Brunner/ Mazel.

Lucas, C. (1964). *Recreation in gerontology.* Springfield, Ill.: Charles C Thomas.

Merritt, M. C. (1971). *Dance therapy program for nursing homes.* Boston: Unitarian University Association.

Mitchell, E. D., & Mason, B. S. (1948). *The theory of play* (rev. ed.). New York: Ronald Press.

Moreno, J. L. (1934). *We shall survive: A new approach to human instruction.* Washington, D.C.: Nervous and Mental Disease Publication Co.

Naumberg, M. (1950). *Schizophrenic art: Its meaning in psychotherapy.* New York: Grune & Stratton.

Nolter, N. (1973). Drama for the elderly: They can do it. *Gerontologist, 13,* 153–156.

Rathbone, J., & Lucas, C. (1970). *Recreation in total rehabilitation* (2nd ed.). Springfield, Ill.: Charles C Thomas.

Rhyne, J. (1973). *The gestalt art experience.* Monterey, Calif.: Brooks/Cole.

Robins, F., & Robins, J. (1965). *Educational rhythmics for mentally handicapped children.* New York: Horizon Press.

Rosen, E. (1957). *Dance in psychotherapy.* New York: Columbia University, Teachers College Bureau Publications.

Roth, E. (1961). Lernen in verschiedenen Altersstufen. *Zeitschrift fuer Experimentelle und Angewandte Psychologie, 8,* 409–417.

Schneider, E. H., Unkefer, R. F., & Gaston, E. T. (1968). Introduction. In E. T. Gaston (Ed.), *Music in therapy* (pp. 1–6). New York: Macmillan.

Shivers, J. S., & Fait, H. F. (1980). *Recreational services for the aged.* Philadelphia, Pa.: Lea & Febiger.

Sunderland, J. T. (1976). *Older Americans and the arts.* Washington, D.C.: National Council on the Aging.

Vorenberg, B. L. (1979). *Enriching an older person's life through senior adult theater.* Unpublished master's thesis, University of Oregon, Eugene, Oreg.

Wadeson, H. (1980). *Art psychotherapy.* New York: John Wiley & Sons.

Wapner, E. B. (1981). *Recreation for the elderly.* New York: Todd & Honeywell.

Way, B. (1967). *Development through drama.* New York: Humanities Press.

Wells, A. (1954). Rhythmic activities on wards of senile patients. In M. Bing (Ed.), *Music therapy* (pp. 127–132). Lawrence, Kans.: Allen Press.

Wells, F. (1977). Psychosonics. In W. Anderson (Ed.), *Therapy and the arts: Tools of consciousness* (pp. 67–82). New York: Harper & Row.

Chapter 10

Managing Tension and Coping with Stress in Late Life

As Pfeiffer (1977) points out, most mental pathology in late life is due to the failure of the older person to cope with the various stresses of late life. In this chapter, we provide a cursory review of the vast literature on factors that mediate the negative effects of stress. This knowledge can help us predict which elderly individuals will effectively cope with stress and which ones will succumb and fall victim to physical or mental illness or, perhaps, even kill themselves. We also review the literature on coping strategies and tension management. Finally, we offer some practical suggestions—derived from the fields of holistic health, recreational therapy, and other relevant fields—that can help provide the troubled elderly with a stress survival kit.

FACTORS MEDIATING THE NEGATIVE EFFECTS OF STRESS

Whether the aging individual effectively withstands stress or succumbs to mental or physical breakdown, death, or suicide depends in large part on the individual's personal resources (health and income), social supports (family, friends, formal and informal group memberships), personality characteristics (ego defenses, flexibility), and coping strategies (fight, flight, freeze). Hamburg, Coehlo, and Adams (1974) have identified four requirements for effective adaptation to stress: (1) containment of distress within tolerable limits, (2) maintenance of self-esteem, (3) preservation of interpersonal relationships, and (4) ability to meet the conditions of the new environment. In developing her model of adaptation to stress, George (1980) suggests that adjustment consists, objectively, of the individual successfully meeting the demands of the environment and, subjectively, of the individual perceiving and experiencing a sense of general well-being in relation to the environment. She asserts that, in the face of crises (such as major role transitions or status changes), the individual strives to maintain a sense of identity and to adjust to new environment demands. Some older people successfully negotiate the challenges of such changes, while others cannot and suffer.

What factors facilitate effective adjustment to change and what circumstances impede successful adjustment? Based on a careful review of existing literature, George (1980) concluded that three factors are involved: personal resources, such as money, education, and health; coping skills; and status characteristics, such as race and sex. In a recent study, Elwell and Maltbie-Crannell (1981) found that income, health, education, and the social support of family and friends significantly lessened the negative impact of stress on their elderly subjects, particularly elderly males. They discovered a strong direct negative relationship between role loss and the personal resources and social support that were available. That is, those who had lost more social roles also had less money, poorer health, and fewer relations with family and friends.

In their large-scale Duke studies, Palmore, Cleveland, Nowlin, Ramm, and Siegler (1979) concluded that stressful life events, such as retirement, do not per se cause problems for the aged; however, those elderly with few psychological, personal, and social resources who suffer many losses in a short period of time are particularly vulnerable to breakdown. The relevant personal and psychological resources included intellectual functioning, personality, and level of anxiety. The social resources included income, education, and density of social network (spouse, children, friends, neighbors, other relatives, and confidants). Along these same lines, Blau (1973) and Lopata (1978) cite the importance of optional role resources and of education, occupation, and social support in facilitating adjustment to the loss of a spouse. Lowenthal et al. (1975) similarly discovered that health and social supports aided adjustment to major role changes in late life.

Social support is a major factor mediating the negative effects of stress and facilitating adjustment to status change and role transition. Lin, Ensel, Simeone, and Kuo (1979) define social support as "support accessible to an individual through social ties to other individuals, groups, and the larger community" (p. 108). Social support is usually derived from family, other relatives, friends, confidants, neighbors, or members of some close-knit support group. Findings from a variety of studies suggest that an intact social support system has a mediating or buffering effect on stress produced by life changes and ill health (Eaton, 1978; Fuller & Larson, 1980; Gelein, 1980; Gore, 1978; Hale & Lebovitz, 1974; Janis, 1974; Nuckolls, 1972; Cassel & Kaplan, 1979; Peznecker & McNeil, 1975). Such a system provides not only unconditional love, caring, and acceptance, but also economic resources, help with the tasks of daily living, and others with whom one can talk and meaningfully share time.

Eisdorfer and Wilkie (1977) found that money was a major factor mediating the negative effect of retirement on males. The amount of preretirement preparation also affected adaptation. Indeed, many studies have identified the positive effects of preretirement preparation in successful adjustment to retirement (Atchley, 1976; Coelho & Adams, 1974; Glamser & DeJong, 1975, Kalt & Kohn, 1975; Palmore, 1982). Atchley (1975) also found that money facilitated adjustment to the loss of a spouse.

In his monumental work on stress, Antonovsky (1979) refers to generalized resistance resources (GRRs). A GRR is "any characteristic of the person or group or the environment that can facilitate effective tension management" (p. 99). Tension management is defined as "the rapidity and completeness with which problems are resolved and tension dissipated" (p. 96). Stress produces tension and, if this tension is not successfully reduced, stress will result in disease or mental or physical ill health. In addition to "avoider" GRRs—such as preventive knowledge, attitudes, and behaviors—Antonovsky lists as GRRs (1) money; (2) cognitive/emotional factors, such as intelligence, knowledge, and ego integrity; (3) value/attitudinal factors, including one's coping strategies; (4) interpersonal relationships and social supports; and (5) macrosociocultural factors, such as one's religious beliefs and the influence of society on the individual. Music is also identified as a GRR. In this regard, Thomas (1974) notes that:

> it is one of our problems that as we become crowded together, the sounds we make to each other become more random-sounding, accidental, or incidental, and we have trouble selecting meaningful sounds out of the noise. . . . We are only saved by music from being overwhelmed by nonsense. . . . The need to make music, and to listen to it is universally expressed by human beings. (pp. 22–24)

One cannot overstate the importance of good health, money, education, occupation, and involvement in support systems as mediators of stress and factors that help older individuals manage tension. Just as important, however, are other more personal characteristics, such as one's philosophy of life—how happy, anxious, or candid one is, how much personal mastery and control one has, and how one personally experiences the aging process.

INTRAPERSONAL RESOURCES AND COPING STRATEGIES

Some individuals are more likely to fall victim to stress than others. The hard-driving go-getter who has inflexible ambitions and is bent on success, achievement, and perfection is in for a hard time when confronted by the losses of late life (failing eyesight and hearing; loss of mobility and health; loss of income, status, and power). On the other hand, the constant worrier who is always anxious and magnifies little things into major earth-shattering events is also in for trouble when the process of aging accelerates. Those who are fearful, guilty, bitter, supersensitive, those who harbor anger, resentment, envy, and hostility, and those who are self-haters and self-blamers are all more likely to fall victim to stress in late life. According to Fiske (1980), those who feel dissatisfaction, disappointment, despair, and disheartenment are likely to experience any loss as a threat to their own integrity and self-esteem rather than as a blow inflicted from the outside over which they have no control. Elderly individuals with good verbal skills, high intelligence, a good memory, high morale, a good self-concept, a sense of mastery or control over life, well-developed psychological defenses, and flexible personalities fare better when confronted by the multiple stresses of aging.

Based on her indepth study of successful adjustment to stress over the life cycle, Fiske (1980) identified the following intrapersonal resources as facilitating successful adjustment: emotional maturity, strength of character, hope, a positive view of life and aging, candidness, gregariousness, a cheerful disposition, a good sense of humor, a sense of ego integrity, a view that one's life has been meaningful and worthy, a sense of inner control, personal affection, autonomy, and a sense of mastery. Those who fared best in the face of life's crises were flexible, creative, and innovative. They anticipated changes and allowed a moratorium for self-repair. They experienced a sense of continuity in goals, interests, and values over the life cycle, and these served as their chief bulwarks against the onslaught of change and conflict (personal and environmental). They tended to be committed to people, to projects, and to certain beliefs. They viewed aging as a challenge and an opportunity and enjoyed deciding how to use their time, talents, resources, and energy. As Fiske (1980) concluded, "For older people who know what they value, what is worth striving for, and how to love, life remains dignified, and death, while perhaps viewed with regret or sadness, holds no terrors, for they have truly lived their lives" (p. 369).

Antonovsky (1979) has emphasized the importance of a sense of personal autonomy and competence to combat the stresses of life. Individuals need a sense that they are in control of their lives, that their internal and external worlds are predictable and controllable. They must be stable and integrated, yet dynamic and flexible. In short, as Stec (1981) notes, "Some people know their own emotional levels. They're neither belligerent nor passive and seem to know when to say no, when to argue the point, and when to give in just a little" (p. 2). Thus, in general, those who have a zest for life, who accentuate the positive, who feel they are in control of their own lives, who are fond of certain people, places, or things, and who have a commitment to beliefs, values, or causes greater than themselves are more likely to adapt successfully to the various stresses of late life.

Many students of stress have focused on personality characteristics and coping strategies that mediate the negative impact of stress. McIntosh, Hubbard, and Santos (1981), Rosow (1973), Miller (1979), and others have stressed the importance of personality and coping style in predicting elderly suicide and reaction to stress. Rosow (1973) suggests that people can be placed on a continuum. On the one end are those who have unusual flexibility and a high tolerance for stress, are resilient, and have personalities that allow them to adjust to strain; on the other end are persons with low tolerance for strain, limited personality resources, and rigid, ineffective modes of responding to crises.

In this context, according to Birren and Renner (1977), personality intervenes in four ways: Behaviorally, some people create or seek stress, others avoid or minimize it; internally, when confronted with stress, some amplify it, others dampen it. Hurst, Jenkins, and Rose (1977) have identified a factor they call "systematic emotional arousal" (p. 415), by which they mean the emotional reaction to stress; that is, some get more upset over a certain life event than do others. Lundberg, Theorell, and Lind (1975) found a considerable difference between those who had suffered a myocardial infarction and those in a control group in the degree of emotion felt regarding a stressful event. Those who had suffered a myocardial infarction tended to attribute more emotional significance to a stressful event and to get more upset over it than did those in the control group.

Atchley (1976) and George (1980) have both noted the importance of flexibility in facilitating successful adaptation to retirement and other events characteristic of late life. The flexible individual can successfully cope with stress by adjusting to new circumstances, by changing patterns of thinking or behavior if necessary, and by taking life as it comes.

Miller (1979) and McIntosh et al. (1981) point out that the coping strategies that can be relied upon in late life are developed early in life and practiced and refined throughout adolescence and mid-life. Similarly, Eisdorfer and Wilkie (1977), George (1980), and Fiske (1980) note the importance of past experience in coping with current situations. Those who have faced stressors in the past and have managed to cope with them do much better in coping with new stresses in late life compared with those who have led fairly stress-free lives earlier and thus have never had to learn to deal with and manage stress.

Coping has been defined as "any response to . . . life strains that serves to prevent, avoid, or control emotional distress" (Perlin & Schooler, 1978, p. 3). Coping encompasses the "covert and overt behaviors which individuals use to prevent, alleviate, or respond to a stressful situation" (George, 1980, p. 30).

Personality, attitudes, beliefs, emotions, psychological defenses, ego strength, and habitual styles of response to specific life conditions and events are all part of coping with the stresses of daily life.

Three late-life coping strategies that have been described in the literature are (1) renewed assault on goals established earlier in life (Janis, 1974); (2) psychological and social denial (Weisman, 1972; Weisman & Hackett, 1967); and (3) "freeze" (Jarvik & Russell, 1977), an adaptive response in which the elderly play dead and shift their mind into neutral. In his classic study of coping and recovery from illness, Janis (1974) found that those who took a problem-focused approach, gathered information, and put up active resistance had the greatest chance of recovery. Cohen (1980), however, found that avoidance and denial strategies worked best for breast cancer patients. Similarly, Felton and Kahana (1974) reported that, for the institutionalized aged, passive coping styles were more effective, and those who did not engage in active assaults on problems were happier and better adjusted. Thus, in certain situations, denial may be the most effective coping strategy; in others, information seeking and active assault on the problem may prove most beneficial. It is important to know when to fight and when to accept the situation. As Selye (1974) puts it, "Fight for your highest attainable aim, but never put up resistance in vain" (p. 12).

Lazarus (1966, 1967, 1968, 1975) and Lazarus, Averill, and Opton (1974) have noted the importance of cognitive processes in coping. Two components of cognitive appraisal are identified: primary appraisal, in which the individual evaluates the person-environment transaction to determine if the event is stressful and, if so, to what extent; and secondary appraisal, in which the individual evaluates coping resources and the options available. Obviously, impaired sight, hearing, or memory and other cognitive impairments negatively affect coping.

Fiske (1980) has identified four types of coping, depending on the level of presumed stress and preoccupation with stress. The *overwhelmed* had had many stressful experiences and dwelt on them at length. The *challenged* similarly had been besieged by stresses in life, but they were not excessively preoccupied with them and spoke little of them. The *self-defeating* had experienced few stressful experiences but dwelt considerably on each one; these were in the "poor me" group. Finally, the *lucky* had experienced few stresses during their lives and were glad of it; they referred to themselves as blessed by God or fate, somehow "protected," and, of the four types, were the least anxious or concerned about death and dying. Thus, cognitive appraisal and emotional state are important determinants of how stressful situations will be perceived, how they will be responded to, and what level of emotion will be aroused in the individual.

Some researchers have turned their attention to the specific coping strategies that the elderly use to manage stress in their lives. Such strategies differ in their degree of rationality, flexibility, farsightedness, and emotional affect (Antonovsky, 1979). Williams and Wirths (1965) have described two basic types of coping styles the elderly use to maintain homeostasis between themselves and their social environment: An autonomous person maintains balance with the environment by more energy output, whereas the dependent person requires more input to maintain balance. In their analysis of reactions to life stress, Thomae and Simons (1967) found that persistent and unavoidable stress situations call for cognitive restructuring rather than ego defense. The individuals who react to stress situations by accurate perception, rather than distortion, are more successful in adapting to the stress than those who do not so react.

Horowitz and Wilner (1980) attempted to delineate particular coping techniques that are effective in combating stress. They developed a coping inventory that they administered to cancer patients and their significant others and also to a group who had come to the clinic for treatment of stress-response syndromes following a serious life event. In their study, they identified three kinds of coping strategies: (1) turning to other attitudes and activities, (2) working through the event, and (3) socialization. They found that the socialization method was the most effective. Talking to friends, finding someone who could offer advice and support and provide direction, and trying to be involved with and useful to others were identified as effective ways to cope with cancer and other traumatic life events. For some, however, the other two strategies were also effective.

Salisbury (1980) reported slightly different results when studying residents aged 60 to 94 in an institution for the aged in New York City. He found that nonsocial or solo activities, such as taking a walk alone, and parasocial activities, such as reading magazines or books or watching television, were reported by the residents as the most effective ways to cope with boredom and loneliness, to forget problems, and to relieve tension. Some did use social strategies or interpersonal contacts; however, these were the least frequently chosen methods of coping. Salisbury suggests an interesting interpretation for his finding that solo activities were the most frequently chosen to relieve boredom and loneliness and release tension. He suggests that not many of the elderly he studied had easily accessible close friends or relatives. He also notes that solo activities allow the elderly to maintain personal control and autonomy and a sense of mastery over time and the environment.

Birren (1969) identified an effective coping strategy that is used particularly by those in middle age. In this age group, those who can systematically construct a "map of life" to guide their actions and help them conserve their energy are the best copers. These individuals can successfully "chunk" information and input from the environment, place it appropriately on the map, and thus reduce their load.

Despite these findings, at this stage of research on stress, coping, and adaptation, we still know very little about the particular defense mechanisms and coping techniques that are most effective in particular situations and under certain conditions. However, the skillful practitioner often can obtain valuable insight about the coping strategies of an individual merely by carefully listening and by asking probing questions. In some cases it may become apparent just from listening to the person that maladaptive defenses and coping strategies are being employed. The task of the caregiver thus becomes one of developing new, more effective coping techniques.

DEVELOPING A PERSONAL STRESS SURVIVAL KIT

Constant fatigue, muscle strains and aches (particularly in the neck and shoulder or lower back area), headaches, eye twitches, and a rapidly beating heart or increased rate of respiration are all symptoms of stress. Practitioners should learn to be aware of these bodily signs of stress in the aged individuals they see; they can alert the practitioner to the fact that the individual is suffering from stress just as quickly and reliably as any checklist or other such measure of stressful life events. In this section, we describe the essential elements of a personal stress survival kit. Unlike some of the social and psychological resources discussed earlier, most of these elements are directly under the control of the older individual. The elements include:

- diet and nutrition
- activity
- exercise
- relaxation
- learning
- leisure competency
- sense of humor
- positive mental attitude and outlook on life

Diet and Nutrition

A well-balanced, nutritious diet is important at any age but it is particularly important in later years because then the body tends to deplete certain vitamins and minerals. Vitamins B and C, iron, potassium, and calcium are the most likely to be lacking (Metress, 1981). Vitamin C is essential to fight off infections and thus helps prevent internal stress from disease. Vitamin B, iron, potassium, and other trace minerals help to mitigate the negative effects of stress and to prevent exhaustion, irritability, and lethargy. The elderly individual should eat citrus fruits, green leafy vegetables, lentils, fish, bananas, brewer's yeast, wheat germ, and whole grains in order to get all of the Vitamin C, B, and minerals needed to avoid or fight stress. At the same time, they should avoid sugars, which interfere with the absorption of potassium, Vitamin C, and B-complex vitamins; caffeine, which destroys the effects of B-complex vitamins and Vitamin C, overstimulates the nervous system, and inhibits the absorption of iron, potassium, silicon, and other trace minerals; alcohol, which also destroys B and C vitamins and puts sugar into the body system; and salt, which drives potassium out of the cells, resulting in exhaustion and lethargy.

Activity

Studies of aging, activity, life satisfaction, self-esteem, and self-concept have convincingly demonstrated the positive effect of high activity levels on morale and self-esteem. Older persons who are active in church activities, political activities, neighborhood clubs and groups, the creative arts, or other personally meaningful activities stand a better chance of remaining interested in life, of being happy, and of feeling good about themselves and their abilities. As Wolff (1970) notes, "The elderly person needs someone or something to live for, to be deeply interested in, to permit him/her happiness and fulfillment. Life has to remain meaningful and purposeful" (p. 73).

Exercise

In addition to its numerous physiological and psychological benefits, exercise plays a major role in stress reduction. Physical exercise provides an outlet for the chemicals produced when the body is prepared for flight or fight during stress. Exercise provides a healthy alternative outlet for the harmful stress chemicals that would otherwise be released into the muscles and bloodstream. Specifically, exercise reoxygenates the blood, helps tighten the muscles, burns up excess sugars and fats, and releases excess energy that might otherwise result in anger or anxiety in the individual (Norfolk, 1976). It usually demands our full concentration and attention, thus diverting our minds from our own troubles and from the daily hassles of living for a brief time. It forces us to become aware of our bodies and to get in touch with how we are feeling and with our muscles, breathing, and heartbeat. Most of us feel better after exercising—calmer, more relaxed, and peaceful—because we have released tension and reduced stress; we can feel the difference.

Relaxation

Being "uptight," nervous, or on edge is usually a sign of being under stress. Exercise is one way to relax, but there are numerous other ways; dancing or just swinging and swaying to some pleasant music, aerobics, doing tai chi exercises, praying, meditating, listening to or playing music, taking a nature walk, sitting in a steamroom or sauna, or taking a long, luxurious bubble bath can all be relaxing. Relaxation in these ways can lower blood pressure (Redmond, Gaylor, McDonald, & Shapiro, 1974); and it has been scientifically demonstrated that those who meditate regularly can withstand more life changes with less illness (Goleman, 1976). Meditation can result in such physiological changes as a lower metabolic rate, reduced oxygen consumption, a decreased heart and respiration rate, and different brain wave patterns. Similarly, some researchers have noted positive physiological and psychological changes derived from prayer (Osborne, 1974). In all these situations, the improved state may be attributed to what Wallace and Benson (1972) call the "relaxation response."

Relaxation, like exercise, is a means of fighting stress. Animal studies conducted at Cornell have revealed that animals that were subjected to continued stress and took several short rest breaks in a day showed fewer ill effects than those animals who did not rest or take a break (Stec, 1981). Thus, those experiencing stress should be encouraged to take several short breaks during their day—for example, by getting out of the room and going outdoors to see a tree, smell a flower, or listen to the birds, or simply by closing one's eyes, taking a few deep breaths, and concentrating on relaxing various muscle systems.

Learning

A study by Northcutt (1978) revealed that, of all age groups, the group aged 60 and over is the least functionally competent, that is, least able to meet successfully the ordinary requirements of daily life in our society. Persons in this age group have the poorest communication, computation, and problem-solving skills and the poorest skills in developing and handling interpersonal relationships. As a result, they have the most problems in such areas of adult living as consumer economics, health, consumer resources, government, and law.

Education and learning are thus important means of providing the elderly individual with the necessary tools to function in our complex society, with the means for self-discovery, creativity, and social involvement. Proper learning with regard to diet, health, and nutrition, to the role of exercise and relaxation in stress reduction, to ways of dealing with the welfare, medical, and legal systems to obtain needed benefits and services, and to the use of leisure time is essential for the elderly individual. Ideally, these skills should be acquired early in life and developed and refined in later years. Still, even those who acquire the needed education in late life are better prepared to cope with their medical, financial, and legal problems and to face the losses they encounter as they age. The relevant learning helps strengthen ego defenses, builds self-concept and self-esteem, and develops flexibility and rationality, and thus can help aged individuals to develop more innovative, creative solutions to their problems. In particular, elderly individuals who are confronted with multiple problems and few solutions should be encouraged to seek means for self-education and formal learning.

Leisure Competency

Most people in our society will spend approximately one third of their lives in leisure, outside of productive employment in the labor force. It is thus essential that the elderly develop leisure competency. Tedrick (1982) suggests that older persons who have achieved leisure competency have clarified their values on the use of discretionary time, have a knowledge of available leisure resources and services, and have developed the skills and appreciations that lead to enjoyment of participation in selected areas. Yet, many of our elderly were raised in an era when hard work was stressed and leisure was denigrated. As a result, they do not have favorable attitudes toward leisure and leisure skills and do not derive pleasure from leisure participation. It thus often becomes necessary to help them develop positive attitudes toward leisure and to assist them in acquiring the knowledge and skills they need to participate in leisure activities.

A Sense of Humor

In the face of all the problems and losses of growing old, it is essential that the elderly maintain their sense of humor. The ability to laugh at one's self and at the events of life eases some of the stresses of living. Older people who feel that life in their later years is not so bad often have a good sense of humor and do not take life or themselves too seriously. They can laugh at life's challenges and relieve their tension in doing so. It is particularly important to encourage humor and laughter in the depressed elderly. Jokes, cartoons, and funny stories can serve the purpose, but a sense of humor about life in general should also be encouraged.

Positive Mental Attitude and Outlook on Life

Among the personal qualities that enable one to age gracefully, R. Gross, B. Gross, and Seidman (1978) listed the following: an intense love of life, the ability to enjoy and give joy, a tendency to look at the positive side of life and find the good in people and events, a deep love and appreciation for beauty and nature, a love of people, and modesty, optimism, and curiosity. Like a good sense of humor, a positive mental attitude and an ability to look at the positive aspects of life and aging are essential ingredients in reducing stress and facilitating the coping process. Thus, practitioners should encourage troubled elderly individuals to see the positive aspects of their lives and of life in general. One way to do this is to encourage them to develop an appreciation for nature, music, and the arts.

REFERENCES

Antonovsky, A. (1979). *Health, stress, and coping.* San Francisco: Jossey-Bass.

Atchley, R. C. (1975). Dimensions of widowhood in later life. *Gerontologist, 15,* 175–178.

Atchley, R. C. (1976). *The sociology of retirement.* New York: John Wiley & Sons.

Birren, J. E. (1969). Age and decision strategies. In A. T. Welford & J. E. Birren (Eds.), *Decision making and age* (pp. 23–26). New York: S. Karger.

Birren, J. E., & Renner, V. J. (1977, April). *Health behavior and aging.* Paper presented at the conference of the Institute de la Vie, Vichy, France.

Blau, Z. S. (1973). *Old age in a changing society.* New York: New Viewpoints.

Coelho, G. V., & Adams, J. E. (1974). Introduction. In G. V. Coelho, D. A. Hamburg, & J. E. Adams (Eds.), *Coping and adaptation* (pp. xv–xxv). New York: Basic Books.

Cohen, F. (1980). Coping with surgery: Information, psychological preparation and recovery. In L. Poon (Ed.), *Aging in the 1980's: Psychological issues* (pp. 375–388). Washington, D.C.: American Psychological Association.

Eaton, W. W. (1978). Life events, social supports, and psychiatric symptoms. *Journal of Health and Social Behavior, 19,* 230–234.

Eisdorfer, C., & Wilkie, F. (1977). Stress, disease, aging, and behavior. In J. E. Birren & K. W. Schaie (Eds.), *Handbook of the psychology of aging* (pp. 251–275). New York: Van Nostrand Reinhold.

Elwell, F., & Maltbie-Crannell, A. D. (1981). The impact of role loss upon coping resources and life satisfaction of the elderly. *Journal of Gerontology, 36,* 223–232.

Felton, B., & Kahana, E. (1974). Adjustment and situationally bound loss of control among institutionalized aged. *Journal of Gerontology, 29,* 295–301.

Fiske, M. (1980). Tasks and crises of the second half of life: The interrelationship of commitment, coping, and adaptation. In J. E. Birren & R. B. Sloane (Eds.), *Handbook of mental health and aging* (pp. 337–376). Englewood Cliffs, N.J.: Prentice-Hall.

Fuller, S. S., & Larson, S. B. (1980). Life events, emotional support, and health of older people. *Research in Nursing and Health, 3,* 81–89.

Gelein, J. L. (1980). The aged American female: Relationships between social support and health. *Journal of Gerontological Nursing, 6,* 69–73.

George, L. K. (1980). *Role transitions in later life.* Monterey, Calif.: Brooks/Cole.

Glamser, F. D., & DeJong, G. F. (1975). The efficacy of preretirement preparation programs for industrial workers. *Journal of Gerontology, 30,* 595–599.

Goleman, D. (1976). Meditation helps break the stress spiral. *Psychology Today, 10,* pp. 82–93.

Gore, S. (1978). The effect of social support in moderating the health consequences of unemployment. *Journal of Health and Social Behavior, 19,* 157–165.

Gross, R., Gross, B., & Seidman, S. (Eds.). (1978). *The new old: Struggling for decent aging.* Garden City, N.Y.: Doubleday.

Hale, S., & Lebovitz, B. D. (1974). *Stress, isolation, and psychiatric impairment among the urban elderly.* Paper presented at the 27th annual meeting of the Gerontological Society of America, Portland, Oreg.

Hamburg, D. A., Coelho, G. V., & Adams, J. E. (1974). Coping and adaptation: Steps toward a synthesis of biological and social perspectives. In G. V. Coelho, D. A. Hamburg, & J. E. Adams (Eds.), *Coping and adaptation* (pp. 403–440). New York: Basic Books.

Horowitz, M. J., & Wilner, N. (1980). Life events, stress, and coping. In L. Poon (Ed.), *Aging in the 1980's: Psychological issues* (pp. 363–374). Washington, D.C.: American Psychological Association.

Hurst, M. W., Jenkins, C. D., & Rose, R. M. (1977). The assessment of life change stress: A comparative and methodological inquiry. *Psychosomatic Medicine, 39,* 413–431.

Janis, I. (1974). Vigilance and decision-making in personal crisis. In G. V. Coelho, D. A. Hamburg, & J. E. Adams (Eds.), *Coping and adaptation* (pp. 139–175). New York: Basic Books.

Jarvik, L. E., & Russell, D. (1977). Anxiety, aging, and the third emergency reaction. *Journal of Gerontology, 34,* 197–200.

Kalt, N. C., & Kohn, M. H. (1975). Pre-retirement counseling: Characteristics of programs and preferences of retirees. *Gerontologist, 15,* 179–181.

Lazarus, R. S. (1966). *Psychological stress and the coping process.* New York: McGraw-Hill.

Lazarus, R. S. (1967). Cognitive and personality factors underlying threat and coping. In M. H. Appley & R. Trumbull (Eds.), *Psychological stress: Issues in research* (pp. 151–169). New York: Appleton-Century-Crofts.

Lazarus, R. S. (1968). Emotions and adaptation: Conceptual and empirical relations. In W. J. Arnold (Ed.), *Nebraska symposium on motivation* (pp. 175–266). Lincoln, Nebr.: University of Nebraska Press.

Lazarus, R. S. (1975). Psychological stress and coping in adaptation and illness. In S. M. Weiss (Ed.), *Proceedings of the National Heart and Lung Institute working conference on health behavior* (DHEW Publication No. 76–868, pp. 51–54). Washington, D.C.: Department of Health, Education, & Welfare.

Lazarus, R. S., Averill, J. R., & Opton, E. M., Jr. (1974). The psychology of coping: Issues of research and assessment. In G. V. Coelho, D. A. Hamburg, & J. E. Adams (Eds.), *Coping and adaptation* (pp. 249–315). New York: Basic Books.

Lin, N., Ensel, W., Simeone, R. & Kuo, W. (1979). Social support, stressful life events, and illness: A model and an empirical test. *Journal of Health and Human Behavior, 20,* 108–119.

Lopata, H. Z. (1978). Contributions of the extended families to the social support systems of metropolitan area widows: Limitations of the modified kin network. *Journal of Marriage and the Family, 40,* 358–364.

Lowenthal, M. F., Thurnher, M., Chiriboga, D. A., & Associates. (1975). *Four stages of life: A comparative study of men and women facing transitions.* San Francisco: Jossey-Bass.

Lundberg, U., Theorell, T., & Lind, E. (1975). Life changes and myocardial infarction: Individual differences in life change scaling. *Journal of Psychosomatic Research, 19,* 27–32.

McIntosh, J. L., Hubbard, R. W., & Santos, J. F. (1981). Suicide among the elderly: A review of issues with case studies. *Journal of Gerontological Social Work, 4*(1), 63–74.

Metress, S. (1981). Nutrition in old age. In C. Kart & B. Manard (Eds.), *Aging in America: Readings in social gerontology* (2nd ed., pp. 189–207). New York: Mayfield.

Miller, M. (1979). *Suicide after sixty: The final alternative.* New York: Springer.

Norfolk, D. (1976). *The habits of health.* New York: St. Martin's Press.

Northcutt, N. (1978). Adult performance level. In C. Klevins (Ed.), *Materials and methods in continuing education* (pp. 273–281). Los Angeles, Calif.: Klevens Publications.

Nuckolls, K. B., Cassel, J., & Kaplan, B. H. (1972). Psychosocial assets, life crisis, and the prognosis of pregnancy. *American Journal of Epidemiology, 95,* 431–441.

Osborne, C. G. (1974). *Prayer and you.* San Antonio, Tex.: Word Books.

Palmore, E. (1982). Preparation for retirement: The impact of preretirement programs on retirement and leisure. In N. J. Osgood (Ed.), *Life after work: Retirement, leisure, recreation, and the elderly* (pp. 330–341). New York: Praeger Press.

Palmore, E., Cleveland, W. P., Nowlin, J. B., Ramm, D., & Siegler, I. C. (1979). Stress and adaptation in later life. *Journal of Gerontology, 34,* 841–851.

Perlin, I. I., & Schooler, C. (1978). The structure of coping. *Journal of Health and Social Behavior, 19,* 2–21.

Pesznecker, B. C., & McNeil, J. (1975). Relationship among health habits, social assets, psychological well-being, life change, and alterations in health status. *Nursing Research, 24,* 442–447.

Pfeiffer, E. (1977). Psychopathology and social pathology. In J. E. Birren & K. W. Schaie (Eds.), *Handbook of the psychology of aging* (pp. 650–671). New York: Van Nostrand Reinhold.

Redmond, D. P., Gaylor, M. S., McDonald, R. H., & Shapiro, A. P. (1974). Blood pressure and heart-rate response to verbal instruction and relaxation in hypertension. *Psychosomatic Medicine, 36,* 285–297.

Rosow, I. (1973). The social context of the aging self. *Gerontologist, 12,* 82–87.

Salisbury, S. (1980, November). *Help me help myself: A case of coping styles for negative affect.* Paper presented at the annual meeting of the Gerontological Society of America, San Diego, Calif.

Selye, H. (1974). *Stress without distress.* New York: New American Library.

Stec, L. F. (1981, May/June). Stress: It can shatter you unless you have a stress survival kit. *Health and Diet Times,* pp. 1–3.

Tedrick, T. (1982). Leisure competency: A goal for aging Americans in the 1980's. In N. J. Osgood (Ed.), *Life after work: Retirement, leisure, recreation, and the elderly* (pp. 315–318). New York: Praeger Press.

Thomae, H., & Simons, H. (1967). Reaktionen auf Belastung-situationen hoeheren Lebensalter. *Zeitschrift fuer Experimentelle und Angewandte Psychologie, 14,* 290–312.

Thomas, L. (1974). *The lives of a cell.* Toronto, Canada: Bantam Books.

Wallace, R. K., & Benson, H. (1972). The physiology of meditation. *Scientific American, 226,* 84–90.

Weisman, A. D. (1972). Common fallacies about dying patients. In A. D. Weisman (Ed.), *Dying and denying: A psychiatric study of terminality* (pp. 23–41). New York: Behavioral Publications.

Weisman, A. D., & Hackett, T. P. (1967). Denial as a social act. In S. Levin & R. T. Kahana (Eds.), *Psychodynamic studies on aging* (pp. 79–110). New York: International Universities Press.

Williams, R. H., & Wirths, C. G. (1965). *Lives through the years.* New York: Atherton.

Wolff, K. (1970). *The emotional rehabilitation of the geriatric patient.* Springfield, Ill.: Charles C Thomas.

Chapter 11

Societal Changes and the Prevention of Elderly Suicide

Though the various assessment techniques and intervention therapies discussed in previous chapters may reduce the rate of suicide among the aged, the prevention of suicide among the elderly may ultimately depend on societal changes—for example, the satisfaction of basic economic needs and the reduction of poverty among the elderly; improved nutrition and health care delivery; improved transportation; more and better psychological and mental health services; more flexible retirement policies, allowances for elderly individuals to continue working, at least part-time; better preparation for retirement; provision of more and safer housing; increased opportunities for meaningful community involvement and social participation through voluntary organizations and social and leisure activities; and more opportunities for the elderly to be workers, teachers, and leaders in our society. Stricter gun control and stricter restraints on the prescription and distribution of potentially lethal addictive drugs, particularly barbiturates, are other societal changes that would benefit the elderly.

THE IMPORTANCE OF EDUCATION

Education is a major key to suicide prevention in late life. Such education, focused on the symptoms of depression and the warning signals of suicide, should involve not only the elderly themselves but also the personnel who serve the elderly and should be included in public education about the elderly and aging.

An important aspect of this education should be concerned with the aging process itself, providing relevant information on diet and nutrition, health and exercise, and ways to cope with role changes of late life. Thus, as Kelly (1982a) suggests, the education process can give "an individual the opportunity to observe, explore, learn about, play with, continue, refine, and master a variety of activities" (p. 207). It can stimulate self-discovery, creativity, and social involvement. Specifically, as many studies have shown, education targeted on the elderly can improve their physical and mental functioning by imparting appropriate values, skills, attitudes, and behaviors; it can help them use their time in meaningful ways; it can enhance their feelings of self-worth, mastery, and competence; it can assist them in coping with changes of late life; it can offer intellectual stimulation, enhance the elderly's performance in volunteer and advocacy roles, and expand their communication skills; and it can help them to develop flexibility to change and to realize their full potential as self-actualizing human beings (Kelly, 1982b; Kleiber, 1982; Klevins, 1978; Knowles & Klevins, 1978; Ward, 1979).

In addition to such general education concerned with the aging process and how to cope with growing older, the elderly need to be educated about depression and suicide. The symptoms of depression and the warning signals of suicide can be recognized by the elderly individual who is properly informed. The elderly should be aware not only of the symptoms of depression and of ways to recognize suicidal thoughts and impulses in themselves, they should also be taught that depression is treatable and that suicide can be prevented. The vulnerable elderly in particular should be educated regarding the kind of help available to them in their community—the psychological and mental health services, the support groups, and other church, community, and social services that can provide aid and guidance.

The media, churches, doctors, nurses, social workers, pharmacists, workers in adult day care centers and other caregivers who come in contact with the aged can all play roles in such education. In this context, the federal government could fund education programs for the aged or offer income tax credits for tuition paid to promote education for the aged. Local churches, community organizations, colleges, and universities could offer their own education programs for the aged. Finally, specially tailored education through the media could do much to widen educational opportunities for the elderly.

Education for Leisure

Aristotle, Socrates, and other Greek philosophers recognized the important connection between leisure, learning, and living. Socrates asserted that "the aim of all education is to teach man to live the good life" (Parker, 1979, p. 62). The good life was a life of leisure, a life devoted to inner growth and development, mental creativity and expansion, and contemplation—the end of which was the achievement of wisdom and the virtues of honesty, freedom, justice, and truth. To improve the prospects of a good life for our elderly citizens, an important first step would be a greater emphasis on leisure education and on preretirement and postretirement education, planning, and counseling.

There is a particularly pressing need for more education on the development of leisure competency. The Society of Park and Recreation Educators defines leisure education as "a process through which individuals acquire the appropriate attitudes, skills, knowledges, and behaviors which allow them to benefit through their leisure choices" (Mobley, 1981, p. 16). Specifically, as noted previously, older persons who have acquired leisure competency have clarified their values on the use of discretionary time, have a knowledge of available leisure resources and services, and have developed skills and appreciations that lead to enjoyment of participation in selected areas (Tedrick, 1982).

In a recent large-scale survey of older adults conducted by the American Association of Retired Persons (1980), older people identified the problem of how to use the increased amount of leisure time as their third most significant problem, following health and finances. Based on their research studies, Cousins (1968), Simpson, Back, and McKinney (1966), and others suggest that many elderly do not participate in leisure not because of a lack of interest but because of a lack of the basic knowledge, skills, and attitudes needed to participate effectively in leisure. Some researchers suggest that, if such leisure competency is not learned by midlife, it never will be (Cousins, 1968; Lambing, 1972; Snow & Havighurst, 1977).

Ward (1979) suggests that our society has done relatively little to promote creative or self-expressive uses of time throughout the life cycle. "Education is geared toward vocational pursuits rather than socialization for life and leisure interests are subsidiary to work and family careers" (p. 253). Moreover, when "entering old age without suitable leisure patterns older people are unprepared to explore new options in using time. Available activities may be shallow and unfulfilling because they are set up for older people or allow them few meaningful roles" (p. 263).

In a similar vein, Mobley (1981) suggests that "our education system has been geared toward teaching one to make a living with correspondingly little effort directed toward teaching one to make a life" (p. 16). He argues that we have too many programs in career education and vocational training with little emphasis on noncareer training and avocational education.

Clearly, by learning the skills and adopting values and attitudes that allow for full and meaningful participation in leisure, a whole new world of self-discovery, creative expression, fun, and enjoyment becomes available to the elderly. Now leisure activities can help fill the void left by lost work and family roles; contribute to better physical and mental health; enhance feelings of self-worth, self-esteem, mastery, and competence; contribute to human growth and development and personal fulfillment; provide rest, relaxation, and diversion; and help to achieve a sense of ego integrity and personal and social integration (Atchley, 1980; Dumazedier, 1967; Erikson, 1950; Havighurst, 1957, 1961; Kaplan, 1979; Kelly, 1978, 1982b; Kleiber & Kelly, 1980). To achieve these goals, more money, resources, and attention must be devoted by our public schools, institutions of higher education, and continuing education programs to the development of leisure skills and attitudes in the early years and through young adulthood and midlife.

Miller (1979) has identified "retirement shock" as a major precipitating factor in suicide of elderly males. Education and preparation for retirement can clearly play important roles in easing the transition from worker to retiree. Indeed, research has documented the positive effects of preretirement training on adjustment to retirement (Atchley, 1976; Glamser & DeJong, 1975; Palmore, 1982; Streib & Schneider, 1971). However, the programs providing such training are still too few, and many of those that exist are poorly designed or inadequately administered. Moreover, there is very little controlled scientific research documenting the long-term effects of such programs and the differential effects of particular techniques of instruction or strategies on various groups (men versus women, blue-collar versus white-collar workers, minorities versus others) (Mangum, 1982; Palmore, 1982; Slover, 1982). One way to remedy currently existing deficiencies would be to allocate more funds to increase the number and scope of preretirement programs and to conduct more research on their methods and long-term effects on adjustment to retirement. In particular, industry has a responsibility to aid in this effort by offering preretirement and postretirement education, planning, and counseling for employees.

Professional Education

Major emphasis should be placed on educating personnel in the health and mental health fields and those in occupations that serve the elderly concerning the process of aging, thereby making them better prepared to meet the needs of the elderly. Medical schools, nursing schools, and other professional schools should include courses about aging in their curricula. Inservice and on-the-job training programs should be offered for practitioners already working in the field. These programs should be focused on dispelling existing myths about aging and the old. Psychologists, psychiatrists, and other caregivers should be provided accurate information in this area so that they no longer view the aged as clinging, dependent, cranky, rigid, unable to change, demanding, or as cases with poor prognoses. More and better education is needed to build a strong field of geropsychology, producing clinicians who are knowledgeable about aging and the aged and who have the clinical skills and techniques needed for working with the aged.

Physicians, clergy, law enforcement personnel, social workers, and other geriatricians need to be educated regarding the symptoms of depression in late life and the clues and warning signs of suicide in the elderly. Graduate and professional schools can play a major role in providing such education. The media can help by providing adequate information to service providers working with elderly clients. Funding from federal, state, and local governments could be used to offset the cost of such education.

Education in the Community

The general public should also become better educated regarding the aging process, particularly with respect to the symptoms of depression and the warning signals of suicide. Old people in this country are rejected, abandoned, and isolated. Such education is essential to break down the negative societal images of aging and eliminate existing stereotypes and discriminatory barriers that impact on the elderly. Indeed, a major media campaign—financed by government, industry, the private sector, or some combination of these—is necessary to change our attitudes about old people in this country, to enable us to see the aged as potentially valuable contributing members of society. Such a campaign could utilize television and radio, mass-circulated cassette tapes and packaged programs, pamphlets and brochures, and a variety of other media devices. Supported by churches, libraries, industry, YWCAs, YMCAs, educational institutions, and other agencies, such a campaign could have an enormous impact by accurately portraying both the stresses and problems of aging and the joys of growing old.

Like the service providers and the elderly, the public needs to be educated particularly about the symptoms of depression and the warning signals of suicide in the aged. When properly informed, family members, friends, and neighbors are in an ideal position to save the life of a potentially suicidal elderly individual. Again, the relevant education could be provided through various media; churches, places of employment, and voluntary organizations could aid in the effort. Specialized lay organizations, such as the Save-a-Life League on the East Coast, could be of particular help in educating the public about suicide among the elderly. Finally, mental hygiene societies could sponsor educational programs in local communities, teaching people how to recognize depression and clues to potential suicide in older individuals.

THE NEED FOR ACCURATE CASE FINDING AND ACTIVE OUTREACH

It is a well-established fact that suicide prevention centers are not utilized by the elderly (Farberow & Moriwaki, 1975; Tuckman, 1970). The vulnerable elderly are also not likely to call social service agencies. More aggressive means of case finding and a more active outreach are needed to reach the lonely, isolated, depressed, or suicide-prone elderly. Such persons must be actively sought, using tips from doctors, pharmacists, staff people at adult day care centers, the clergy, the police, and others who come in contact with them. Health departments, welfare offices, social security offices, and geriatric screening programs can also provide relevant leads and information. McIntosh, Hubbard, and Santos (1981) suggest establishing separate hot lines for the elderly; setting up special centers to reach the troubled elderly; using other seniors in a sort of "buddy system" to reach those who are vulnerable; and establishing community-based outreach programs to find the suicide-prone elderly. In all these efforts, early case finding is a key to suicide prevention.

There is a clear need for more community-based geriatric services. Such services should actively seek out the troubled elderly. They should also be easily accessible and available to the aged. Their staff should be well-trained in geropsychology, and older individuals should be made available as staff members. Similarly, peer support groups, grief counselors, reminiscence groups, and psychotherapeutic services (individual and group) should be made affordable and available to elderly individuals with problems. After a suicide-prone elderly person is identified and crisis intervention techniques have eliminated any immediate danger of suicide, a program of long-term treatment should be implemented to increase self-confidence and self-esteem, improve communication skills, and reduce isolation. The need for active follow-up in such cases is crucial; periodic assessment of lethality is essential.

CONCLUSIONS

In the final analysis, old people in America kill themselves because old age has nothing worthwhile to offer them (Miller, 1979). As long as we phase our old people out by rejecting them and depriving them of those things that provide meaning and purpose to life at any age—work, community involvement, social relationships, and service—the frequency of suicide will remain high in this age group. As Sainsbury (1962) concluded, "Old people will continue to feel a useless burden and therefore be suicide-prone, until they have a real place in the community" (pp. 168–169). We thus have a clear responsibility either to provide new, meaningful social roles for our elderly or to allow them to continue to perform roles from their earlier years.

As long as we view the aged as useless, nonproductive people to be pitied and feared—perhaps because we see them as living portraits of what we will become if we live long enough—the elderly suicide rate will remain high. Only when old age comes to be viewed once again as a valued status, rather than a cursed disease or burden in our society, will we significantly reduce the number of elderly suicides. Ultimately our aim must be to make the words of Robert Browning a reality in the lives of our elderly:

> Grow old along with me!
> The best is yet to be,
> The last of life, for which the first was made:
> Our times are in His hand
> Who saith "A whole I planned,
> Youth shows but half; trust God:
> See all nor be afraid!
>
> *Rabbi Ben Ezra*

REFERENCES

American Association of Retired Persons. (1980). *Rank order of retirement problems.* Unpublished report, Andrus Gerontology Center, Los Angeles, Calif.

Atchley, R. C. (1976). *The sociology of retirement.* New York: Schenkman.

Atchley, R. C. (1980). *The social forces in later life* (3rd. ed.). Belmont, Calif.: Wadsworth.

Cousins, A. (1968, April 20). Art, adrenalin, and the enjoyment of living. *Saturday Review*, pp. 20–24.

Dumazedier, J. (1967). *Toward a society of leisure.* New York: Collier-Macmillan.

Erikson, E. (1950). *Childhood and society* (2nd ed.). New York: W. W. Norton.

Farberow, N. L., & Moriwaki, S. (1975). Self-destructive crises in the older person. *Gerontologist*, *15*, 333–337.

Glamser, F., & DeJong, G. (1975). The efficacy of preretirement preparation programs for industrial workers. *Journal of Gerontology*, *30*, 595–600.

Havighurst, R. J. (1957). The leisure activities of the middle aged. *American Journal of Sociology*, *63*, 152–162.

Havighurst, R. J. (1961). The nature and value of meaningful freetime activity. In R. Kleemier (Ed.), *Aging and leisure* (pp. 309–344). New York: Oxford University Press.

Kaplan, M. (1979). *Leisure: Lifestyle and lifespan.* Philadelphia: Saunders.

Kelly, J. R. (1978). Situational and social factors in leisure decisions. *Pacific Sociological Review*, *21*, 187–207.

Kelly, J. R. (1982a). *Leisure.* Englewood Cliffs, N.J.: Prentice-Hall.

Kelly, J. R. (1982b). Leisure in later life: Roles and identities. In N. J. Osgood (Ed.), *Life after work: Retirement, leisure, recreation, and the elderly* (pp. 268–292). New York: Praeger Press.

Kleiber, D. (1982). Optimizing retirement through lifelong learning and leisure education. In N. J. Osgood (Ed.), *Life after work: Retirement, leisure, recreation, and the elderly* (pp. 319–329). New York: Praeger Press.

Kleiber, D., & Kelly, J. R. (1980). Leisure socialization and the life cycle. In S. E. Iso-Ahola (Ed.), *Social psychological perspectives on leisure and recreation* (pp. 91–133). Springfield, Ill.: Charles C Thomas.

Klevins, C. (Ed.). (1978). *Materials and methods in continuing education.* Los Angeles: Klevens Publications.

Knowles, M., & Klevins, C. (1978). History and philosophy of continuing education. In C. Klevins (Ed.), *Materials and methods in continuing education* (pp. 8–17). Los Angeles: Klevens Publications.

Lambing, M. L. B. (1972). Leisure time pursuits among retired blacks by social status. *Gerontologist, 12,* 363–367.

Mangum, W. P. (1982). Retirement and leisure: A life course perspective. In N. J. Osgood (Ed.), *Life after work: Retirement, leisure, recreation, and the elderly* (pp. 295–314). New York: Praeger Press.

McIntosh, J. L., Hubbard, R. W., & Santos, J. F. (1981). Suicide among the elderly: A review of issues with case studies. *Journal of Gerontological Social Work, 4*(1), 63–74.

Mobley, T. A. (1981). Leisure counseling: A new profession. *Phi Kappa Phi, 62,* 16–17.

Miller, M. (1979). *Suicide after sixty: The final alternative.* New York: Springer.

Palmore, E. (1982). Preparation for retirement: The impact of preretirement programs on retirement and leisure. In N. J. Osgood (Ed.), *Life after work: Retirement, leisure, recreation, and the elderly* (pp. 330–341). New York: Praeger Press.

Parker, M. (1979). Socrates: The wisest and most just? *Translation from Greek and Roman Authors.* Cambridge, Mass.: Cambridge University Press.

Sainsbury, P. (1962). Suicide in later life. *Gerontologica Clinica, 4*(3), 161–170.

Simpson, I., Back, K., & McKinney, J. (1966). *Social aspects of aging.* Durham N.C.: Duke University Press.

Slover, D. (1982). Preparation for retirement: The impact of preretirement programs. In N. J. Osgood (Ed.), *Life after work: Retirement, leisure, recreation, and the elderly* (pp. 342–350). New York: Praeger Press.

Snow, R., & Havighurst, R. (1977). Life style types and patterns of retirement of educators. *Gerontologist, 17,* 545–552.

Streib, G., & Schneider, C. (1971). *Retirement in American society.* Ithaca, N.Y.: Cornell University Press.

Tedrick, T. (1982). Leisure competency: A goal for aging Americans in the 1980's. In N. J. Osgood (Ed.), *Life after work: Retirement, leisure, recreation, and the elderly* (pp. 315–318). New York: Praeger Press.

Tuckman, J. (1970). Suicide and the suicide prevention center. In K. Wolff (Ed.), *Patterns of self-destruction: Depression and suicide* (pp. 18–28). Springfield, Ill.: Charles C Thomas.

Ward, R. (1979). *The aging experience.* New York: Lippincott.

Index

About the Author

Nancy J. Osgood is Assistant Professor of Gerontology and Sociology at Virginia Commonwealth University/Medical College of Virginia in Richmond. A former member of the National Committee on Vital and Health Statistics, Dr Osgood has interests that include health and mental health of the aged. She has written several papers and articles on the topic of elderly suicide. Her other interests center around the issues of retirement, widowhood, and the impact of various environments on the elderly. Dr. Osgood recently completed *Life After Work: Retirement, Leisure, Recreation, and the Elderly* and *Senior Settlers: Social Integration in Retirement Communities,* both published by Praeger Publishers. With Patch Clark, she is presently completing *Seniors on Stage: The Impact of Creative Dramatics on the Elderly,* to be published by Praeger Publishers. Dr. Osgood teaches classes in recreation, leisure, and aging; community services for the elderly; and social gerontology. Her Ph.D. in sociology and a certificate in gerontology were earned at Syracuse University in 1979.